Gaspar Maximilian Gabriel Morey-Klapsing

Stabilisation of the foot and ankle complex: proactive and reactive responses to disturbances in the frontal plane

SPORT & BUCH *Strauß* – **Köln**

*Schriften zur Biomechanik
des muskulo-skelettalen Systems*

Herausgegeben von Gert-Peter Brüggemann – Köln

*Collected works on the biomechanics
of the musculoskeletal system*

This thesis was accepted by the German Sport University of Cologne as doctoral thesis for obtaining the degree of a PhD in Biomechanics. President of the doctorate committee: Prof. Dr. Ilse Hartmann-Tews. First referee: PD Dr. Adamantios Arampatzis. Second referee: Prof. Dr. Gert-Peter Brüggemann
The thesis was defended on June 16th 2005 at the German Sport University of Cologne

Bibliographic information of the German Bibliotheca

The German Bibliotheca has catalogued this publication in the German national bibliography. Detailed bibliographic data can be found via internet at <http://dnb.ddb.de>

Morey-Klapsing, Gaspar Maximilian Gabriel:
Stabilisation of the foot and ankle complex: proactive and reactive responses to disturbances in the frontal plane
Sport und Buch Strauss, Cologne 2005 – 1st. Edition
ISBN 3-89001-605-7

© Verlag SPORT und BUCH Strauß
Olympiaweg 1 – 50933 Köln
Tel. (02 21) 9 47 21 65
Fax (02 21) 9 47 21 66
e-Mail: verlag@sport-und-buch.de
http://www.sport-und-buch.de
Cover design: Mike Hopf
Print: buch bücher dd ag, Birkach
Printed in Germany

Abstract

This thesis comprises four studies all committed to a better understanding on how functional joint stabilisation is achieved. In order to do so the neuromechanical behaviour of the foot and ankle complex was experimentally studied under different conditions. The first study focused on EMG onset times in response to sudden expected and unexpected tilts, as onset times have been often studied in relation to functional ankle instability and the literature reports controversial results. We found onset time determination to have several inherent methodological problems. In addition their relevance with regard to joint stability remains unclear. Consequently onset times were not considered in the following three studies.

The methods were similar among the remaining studies. The kinematics were determined by means of a three dimensional model of the foot and ankle comprising 4 segments (shank, rearfoot, lateral forefoot column and medial forefoot column). This allowed a more detailed and functional analysis of foot motion, which is an important issue because observing only one of the foot joints does not allow to predict the behaviour of the others. The electromyographic (EMG) signals from six leg muscles as well as the three dimensional ground reaction forces (GRF) were also analysed.

The second study, where expected and unexpected sudden tilts were compared, showed that expectedness could improve joint stabilisation in that the same kinematics and lower GRF were achieved with lower EMG amplitudes. As no differences were observed immediately prior to plate release, it can be stated that the enhanced stabilisation observed for expected trials had to arise from supraspinal influences.

The third study observed sudden unexpected tilts in lateral or medial direction (direction was known). Direction specific as well as common responses to the tilts could be observed in most parameters. Higher mediolateral ground reaction forces and reduced kinematics with no general increase in muscular activation were observed for the medial tilts. This suggests, that passive structures may counteract destabilising forces and this way reduce the otherwise needed muscular activation.

The fourth study dealt with a more functional task: Landings from 40 cm height onto three surfaces with different frontal plane inclination. Contrary to the previous studies, where it was tried to keep the initial conditions identical until plate release, this time also adjustments made prior to the perturbation (ground contact) could be analysed. The results revealed specific adjustments in foot motion and EMG prior to touchdown which were necessarily planned before touchdown. Early specific post-touchdown responses not related to any feedback arising from the collision with the surface were also observed. It is suggested that these are mainly due to self-stabilizing mechanisms of the musculoskeletal system. It was concluded, that different central motor commands were produced in response to the different surfaces. It was hypothesised that the aim of these adjustments is to enhance the self-stabilising potential of the involved structures.

Analysing the results from all four studies together, evidence arises, that stabilisation is mainly achieved by mechanisms others than direct proprioceptive feedback of the acute perturbation. These mechanisms involve prediction of the perturbation to come and passive mechanics.

Acknowledgements

From the academic point of view, which for the last years I could not really separate from my private life, and in chronological order, I would like to thank the people at the IBV (Institut de Biomecànica de València) where I really enjoyed my first steps in the field of biomechanical research. Ilona Gerling built the bridge for me to come over to the German Sport University of Cologne. Prof. Brüggemann opened the doors of his lab to me and shared his enthusiasm on biomechanics and a few of the millions of ideas crossing his head. Dr. Arampatzis tutored me and was my constant scientific guide and conscience during my research activities.

And the colleagues? Of course, the colleagues. Especial thanks go to Dr. Uwe Kersting and Dr. Toni Arndt who took me by the hand during my first steps in Cologne (not only in the lab). Dr. Mark Walsh shared countless hours sitting on the same desk with me ("mucho trabajo, poco dinero"). Gianpiero De Monte was a great help during my measurements and for calming the yearn for mediterranean communication ("tante parole che qui non posso scrivere"). Especial thanks go also to Lida Mademli for checking, re-checking, re-re-checking ... the whole text for typos, format congruence, etc.

Finally I want to thank everyone supporting me during these years: Thank you for your caring help and for being there.

Dedication

To my parents…

…who always let me go and do whatever I thought to be right, supported me in doing it and always kept their arms open for me to come back or hold me when ever it was necessary.

Contents

Prologue 9
Introduction and outline 11

1	First Study: Onset times and joint stabilisation	17
1.1	Introduction	18
1.2	Methods	20
1.3	Results	23
1.4	Discussion	26
1.5	References	29
2	Second Study: Joint stabilising response to expected and unexpected tilts	33
2.1	Introduction	36
2.2	Methods	37
2.3	Results	44
2.4	Discussion	48
2.5	Conclusions	51
2.6	References	51
3	Third Study: Joint stabilising response to lateral and medial tilts	55
3.1	Introduction	56
3.2	Methods	58
3.3	Results	64
3.4	Discussion	69
3.5	Conclusions	71
3.6	References	71

4	Fourth Study: Foot and ankle stabilisation during drop landing: A kinematic, kinetic and electromyographic study	75
4.1	Introduction	76
4.2	Methods	79
4.3	Results	84
4.4	Discussion	91
4.5	References	96

Summary and Conclusions ... 101

Bibliography ... 105

Curriculum Vitae ... 113

Prologue

At the very beginning of my PhD studies, I was supposed to investigate how the muscles of the lower leg control landing and jumping tasks and how this control could influence the storage and delivery of mechanical energy in the foot structures. Special attention should be paid to joint stability and to frontal plane foot motion. One of my first duties was to find out how to classify stable and unstable subjects. Therefore I needed a definition of joint stability. After intensive searching through the literature and consulting experts, I realised that there was no definition suited to my purpose. The nature and the factors affecting joint stability are too manifold. Any objective grouping criterion would describe only a minor aspect of joint stabilisation. The relationship between functional joint stability and classical clinical tests aiming to quantify the degree of mechanical stability (e.g. stress radiography) proved to be low. Finally I had read and thought a lot about the function and the stabilisation of the foot and the ankle complex. It became clear to me that the issue of joint stabilisation is far away from being well understood. So at the end it was decided to try to provide some more insight into this phenomenon. As the famous German tale writer Michael Ende would have said: The issue on the storage and delivery of mechanical energy in the foot and ankle complex is now "another story and shall be told another time".

In the following, four studies concerned with foot and ankle stabilisation are exposed. As each study is intended to be a stand-alone report, many of the methods, the exposed ideas and conclusions are repeated. However each study provides new knowledge and enlightens the issue of joint stabilisation of the foot and ankle complex a bit further. The first three studies are published or in press. You will find some differences among studies in the nomenclature albeit describing the same thing. This is due to the different referees reviewing each study, who exhorted me to do so. The articles are presented as they are published except for the formatting which has been unified throughout the thesis.

Introduction and outline

This thesis focuses on the foot and ankle complex and its stabilisation. There is a reasonable amount of studies done under passive conditions using anatomical preparations (Cass et al., 1984, Siegler et al., 1994) or done with living subjects (Seligson et al., 1980; Liu et al., 2000). These studies provided information regarding the mechanical constraints of foot motion and concentrated almost exclusively on the tibio-talar and the talo-crural joints. Another considerable amount of studies oriented their efforts to elucidate the effectiveness of different orthoses or tape in preventing excessive ankle motion or injuries and to their possible interference with performance (Karlsson and Andreasson, 1992; Eils and Rosenbaum, 2003; Leanderson et al., 1999). In these studies the kinematics were often disregarded or analysed with very simple two-dimensional models. Furthermore again attention was paid only to the tibio-talar and the talo-crural joints, whereas forefoot motion has not been considered. In general the effectiveness of orthoses, at least in reducing the amount of recidives, is supported (Verhagen et al., 2000; Tropp et al., 1985). Other studies tried to identify factors associated to functional ankle instability, i.e. factors favouring recurrent sprains (Neely, 1998; Karlsson et al., 1997). Some of the studied factors have been: **a)** Mechanical instability, which has proven to be associated to functional instability. However the correlation is weak and it is not possible to estimate the degree of the one from the other (Tropp et al., 1985; Vaes et al., 2001). **b)** Latency times, especially of the peroneal muscles. The results from the literature are controversial and somewhat more recently their clinical relevance regarding joint stabilisation has been also questioned (Benesch et al., 2000; Morey et al., 2004). **c)** Joint position sense which seems to be impaired in recurrently sprained ankles (Konradsen et al., 1998; Konradsen, 2002) and **d)** Muscle strength. The results from the literature are differing and not conclusive (Kaminski and Hartsell, 2002; Konradsen et al., 1998).

In contrast to the relatively high amount of literature related to factors associated to functional instability, there is a lack of articles focusing on the understanding on how stabilisation is achieved. One main shortcoming of the existing literature is the use of too simple foot and ankle models, mainly considering the foot as one single segment and observing only one plane of motion. Two studies stressing the importance of forefoot motion, especially in the frontal plane are those from Stacoff et al. (2000) and Arampatzis et al. (2002). One further limitation of most studies in this field is the segmented approach contemplating either neural phenomena or mechanical ones, but not integrating them (Caster and Bates, 1995; Nielsen, 2004). As all factors are interdependent, when observing only one parameter and trying to provide an explanation of the results, the need to rely on assumptions is relatively high. This is because the other involved parameters are not known and their behaviour can at best be only indirectly inferred.

Basing on this background, the present thesis tries to enlighten the topic of joint stabilisation. In order to do this, different stabilisation tasks are studied by measuring their three-dimensional kinematics, not only between rearfoot and the lower leg, but also between the lateral and medial forefoot columns and the rearfoot. This is done by means of a three-dimensional multi-body system model of the shank and the foot (Arampatzis et al., 2002). In addition the activation patterns of six muscles of the lower leg (mm. peroneus longus and brevis, m. tibialis anterior and the three heads of the triceps surae: gastrocnemius lateralis, gastrocnemius medialis and soleus) are estimated using surface electromyography (EMG) and also the three-dimensional ground reaction forces are measured and analysed. Rather than trying to identify factors related to joint instability, this thesis aims to improve our understanding on how joint stabilisation is achieved.

The thesis comprises four studies. Three of them utilise sudden tilt tests in their experimental protocol, whereas the last one focuses on landings. The first study is a critical analysis of the use of EMG onset times with regard to joint stabilisation studies, as this is one of the most utilised approaches. In the three following studies different stabilising demands are experimentally induced. The stabilising responses are then analysed with regard to: the kinematics of the foot and ankle complex, the corresponding EMG signals and the ground reaction forces.

More concisely, in the first study the issue of EMG onset times is critically discussed in their relation to joint stability based on experimental data obtained during tilt plate tests, which represent a typical approach in the field of joint stabilisation studies. Several methodological concerns in their determination are exposed. Furthermore onset times calculated using different algorithms are compared to integrals of the EMG signal regarding their robustness. The information provided by both parameters is discussed. In general the onset times showed a considerably lower repeatability than EMG integrals. In some cases earlier onset times corresponded to lower EMG integrals and in others constant onsets to variable integrals. It is concluded that in many cases onset times alone are not sufficient for describing early muscle activation and when not aware of the limitations, such studies might even induce to misleading conclusions. The additional calculation of amplitude related EMG parameters can provide relevant information regarding the quality of this early activation period.

In the second study the focus is set on the influence of awareness on the response to a sudden inverting tilt. It was assumed that awareness of the instant of tilt would enhance joint stabilisation. The aim was to observe how this advantage is reflected in the considered parameters (kinematics, EMG and ground reaction forces). The kinematics themselves are of interest, since in the literature the information on the kinematics during tilt tests is almost completely restricted to the motion between rearfoot and tibia. At the presented tilt test studies the kinematics are analysed only in the eversion inversion motion of the three modelled joints. This is enough for the purpose of the experiments because the experimental treatment (perturbation) is in this plane of motion and therefore the main effects should also appear in this plane. Whereas unexpected and expected trials did not show significant differences in the kinematics, higher EMG amplitudes and horizontal force amplitudes were found for the unexpected trials. Opposite to that, whereas no differences in electromyographic or ground reaction force parameters were found between stable and unstable subjects (subjective feeling of stability), the kinematics revealed higher amplitudes and velocities for the stable group. It was concluded that awareness can enhance joint stabilisation. The results provide evidence on that this enhancement is triggered at supraspinal levels, as there were no significant differences in any studied parameter prior to plate release, and the only difference between the experimental conditions was the awareness of the instant of tilt. One further conclusion of this study is that higher rather than earlier activation seems to be decisive in joint stabilisation.

In the third study inverting tilts are compared to everting ones. The followed philosophy is similar to that in the second study. This time the perturbations are identical in magnitude but opposite in direction. This protocol aimed to produce generic and specific responses to sudden perturbations of joint position. These should be analysed in all considered parameters (kinematics, EMG and ground reaction forces). Forefoot to rearfoot motion was found to be faster and have greater amplitudes than ankle motion. In general medial tilts showed lower motion amplitudes and angular velocities than lateral tilts but higher horizontal ground reaction force integrals. Interestingly, despite of opposite tilt directions, the EMG patterns were similar for both conditions, indicating that the temporal characteristics of the EMG triggered by joint position perturbations correspond to generic responses which are not, or only weakly related to the direction of the perturbation. The EMG responses showed also some direction specific differences in the amplitudes. The higher mediolateral ground reaction forces, together with the reduced kinematics and no general increase in muscular activation during medial tilts suggest that in this direction the contribution of passive structures to counteract the destabilising forces is higher and sufficient to reduce the otherwise needed muscular activation. This provides evidence on that the contribution of passive structures to joint stabilisation can vary depending on the geometry of the joints and the destabilising forces.

The fourth study, which deals with foot and ankle stabilisation during landings, aimed to examine a more functional task than sudden tilts during quiet standing. Landings are a good model for the study of joint stabilisation (Duncan and McDonagh, 2000; Pelland and McKinley, 2004). Whereas at the former studies of this thesis using tilt plate tests it was tried to keep the initial conditions identical until the instant of the perturbation, at this study the initiation of the fall is controlled, but during the fall there is time to prepare the collision with the ground. This allows changing the orientation of the segments and the activation of the muscles prior to the perturbation (collision). Similar to both former studies the responses of the considered parameters to three different surface conditions (level surface or 3° inclined either medially or laterally) are analysed and compared. Surface specific responses were observed in the kinematics and in the EMG even prior to touchdown, e.g. higher lateral forefoot inversion and peroneal activity for trials onto the laterally inclined surface. The specificity of the response was higher for both forefoot joints than for the ankle joint, especially in eversion-inversion. Similarily the peroneal muscles were more sensitive to surface inclination than the muscles of the triceps surae. The medially inclined surface led to lower mediolateral ground reaction forces near touchdown, and to a lower vertical force maximum than the laterally inclined surface. All these results indicate that early post-touchdown responses can be explained by self-stabilising mechanisms of the musculoskeletal system which are not related to any feedback arising from the collision with the ground. From this study it is concluded, that changes in surface condition can produce different central motor commands. It is suggested that these motor commands aim to enhance the self-stabilising potential of the whole system. This way the need to rely on the relatively slow feedback mechanisms is reduced and the neuromuscular system is relieved. Finally this interpretation of the data, provides a frame which allows explaining the mechanisms behind the success of proprioceptive training in reducing recurrent injuries (Tropp et al., 1985 and 1988; Lephart et al., 1997; Verhagen et al., 2000), without the need to assume that joint stabilisation is largely dependent on proprioception.

1 First Study:
Onset times and joint stabilisation

In most of our joints, an adequate muscle activity is necessary to maintain stability. So muscle activity is one of the important factors to account for when studying joint stabilisation. A considerable amount of research has been done on the field of functional joint stabilisation. Cohen and Cohen (1956) proposed the 'arthrokinetik reflex' as a joint stabilising mechanism. Somewhat later Freeman (1965) stated "functional instability is usually in first place due to incoordination consequent to deafferentiation". Proprioception became a main focus of attention in joint stability studies. In this context, muscle onset times in response to sudden perturbations were considered to be an indicator of proprioceptive performance (Konradsen and Ravn, 1990; Löfvenberg et al., 1995). During the analysis of the literature concerned with joint stability many articles focusing on EMG onset times were found. However, our experience at the institute was that onset times were quite variable. In contrast the amplitude or frequency related parameters were usually far more reliable, even during the pre-innervation phase. This motivated the following study, where several EMG onset detection algorithms were tested and compared to a commonly utilised EMG amplitude related parameter (the integrated EMG).

CHOOSING EMG PARAMETERS:
Comparison of different onset determination algorithms and EMG integrals in a joint stability study

Gaspar Morey-Klapsing
Adamantios Arampatzis
Gert Peter Brüggemann

Institute for Biomechanics,
German Sport University Cologne, Cologne, Germany

Published in:
Clinical Biomechanics (Bristol, Avon). 2004 Feb;19(2):196-201
doi:10.1016/j.clinbiomech.2003.10.010

Abstract

Objective. The aim was to test various algorithms for onset determination and compare onset repeatability to that from integrals of the EMG signal. The information contained in both parameters is discussed.

Design. Onset times were calculated using six different algorithms. The integral of the EMG signal was calculated for seven intervals: From tilt start and from each of the resulting onsets to 200 ms after tilt start.

Background. EMG onset times are often utilised, especially regarding co-ordination patterns or joint stability. There are almost as many different procedures for onset determination as authors dealing with it. Results in the literature are contradictory. The determination and usage of onset times remains controversial.

Methods. EMG signals from 6 muscles of the lower leg of 23 subjects were recorded during three consecutive, expected and unexpected sudden inversion and eversion trials while standing on a tilting platform.

Results. In most cases the repeatability of the onset times was considerably lower than that of the integrals of the EMG for all studied algorithms. In some cases earlier onset times corresponded to lower integral values and constant onsets to variable integrals.

Conclusions. In many cases onset times alone are not sufficient for describing onset phenomena. The additional calculation of the integrated EMG might provide relevant information regarding the quality of early activation.

Relevance

The findings are evidencing that care should be taken when interpreting onset times alone. The additional use of the integral of the EMG signal is suggested to provide more meaningful information.

1.1 Introduction

Muscle onset times are often utilised in studies concerned with electromyography (EMG), most of them regarding co-ordination patterns or joint stability. In the literature we find pure visual determination protocols (Ebig et al., 1997 and Hodges and Bui, 1996), computer aided protocols at which the experimenter has to decide whether or not to accept the detected onset or where to finally place it (Hodges and Bui, 1996 and Di Fabio, 1997), as well as fully automated algorithms (see table 1.1). Different filters and onset thresholds are used and as stated by Hodges and Bui (1996) in many cases the criteria or methods for onset determination are not even specified. Sometimes a fixed value is used as threshold (Zhou et al.,1995), but in most algorithms the threshold is based on the standard deviation or a percentage of the EMG signal while the corresponding muscle is relaxed. As indicated by Winter (1984), the chosen threshold strongly influences the instant of onset detection. Further, the quality of onset time detection strongly depends on the quality of the signal. The fact of having a broad variety of methods (Table 1.1) and the lack of consensus might indicate that none of the known techniques is really satisfactory nor generally accepted. Benesch et al. (2000) despite stating that peroneal reaction time is a stable and reliable parameter, further state that its clinical relevance is not yet clear. So the determination and usage of onset times remains a controversial topic. It is very difficult to differentiate the real variability of a parameter from the variability due to flaws in the detection algorithm (Tomberg et al., 1991). However, making some assumptions, it is possible to estimate the contribution of different sources to the total variability (Brinckmann et al., 2002). Bonato et al. (1988) developed a statistical method using a double threshold detector. This method yields standard deviations below 15 ms when analysing gait patterns. This is enough for many applications and may reflect a real variability. However it is still too much for many other applications, e.g. studies dealing with EMG latency times in response to sudden tilts, where the reported differences between groups are often in the range or below this standard deviation.

The integrated EMG (IEMG) is frequently used for describing EMG activity. There is little, if any, controversy about its use. Further, many studies have dealt with its reliability (Gollhofer et al., 1990; Mero and Komi, 1986; Goodwin et al., 1999; Yang and Winter, 1983). Most of them reporting high correlation values for repeated measures.

To be useful, a parameter should provide relevant information and should be reliable. Onset times have been used for analysing proprioception, but when studying joint stability, the amount of early activity might be crucial and not always related to the onset time. It is hypothesised that: a. onset time detection produces very variable results whereas the calculation of IEMG provides a higher repeatability and b. onset times and IEMG are not necessarily related to each other. Therefore the aims of

Table 1.1. Several authors and the corresponding methods for onset determination used.

Author	Year	Onset determination
Tomberg et al.	1991	Electronic determination by a manually adjusted threshold
McKinley & Pedotti	1992	At above 95% confidence interval for baseline during more than 10 ms
Johnson & Johnson	1993	At 200% above noise
Zhou et al.	1995	At 0.015 mV above baseline value
Lynch et al.	1996	10 SD above lowest rest level in several 100 ms RMS of 200 ms resting EMG
Ebig et al.	1997	Visual determination
Bonato et al.	1998	A statistical method using a double threshold detector
Duncan & McDonagh	2000	Average of the ten highest data points in a fixed window (35–80 ms)
Vaes et al.	2001	At amplitude twice the peak to peak amplitude of average signal noise

this study were: a. to test the reproducibility of several onset determination algorithms and compare it to that from the IEMG and b. expose and compare the information provided by these parameters.

1.2 Methods

The EMG signals (1000 Hz) from 23 subjects (12 males, 11 females; 13 stable, 10 unstable) were recorded using bipolar, pre-amplified surface EMG electrodes placed over the belly of six muscles of the lower leg (peroneus longus, peroneus brevis, soleus, gastrocnemius lateralis, gastrocnemius medialis and tibialis anterior) with an interelectrode distance of 2 cm. The grouping criterion was the subjective feeling of ankle/foot stability as determined by a short anamnestic questionnaire including among others frequency, kind and consequences of inversion trauma. Stable and unstable subjects were analysed separately, since stability could affect the results (Lynch et al., 1996; Vaes et al., 2001). The subjects underwent expected and unexpected sudden inversion and eversion trials (20°) while standing on a tilting platform. The subjects had bare feet and were aware of the tilting direction. Their left leg was full weight bearing, having its longitudinal axis parallel to the tilt axis of the plate. The tip of the right foot rested on a block to help maintain balance (Figure 1.1). The subjects were instructed to look forward to a spot on the wall. The plate was released from behind the subjects out of their field of view. Each subject performed three trials per condition. The instant of release was indicated by counting backwards 3, 2, 1, tilt. At those trials randomly chosen to be unexpected the plate was released at any time during the countdown. The first trial of each condition was always unexpected. The onset times were determined using an algorithm with 6 different parameter combinations (Table 1.2). It was defined as the time between start of the tilt, as determined by an electrogoniometer (1000 Hz) aligned with the axis of rotation of the tilt plate, and the instant at which the filtered signal exceeded the given threshold. Two different median filters, window widths of 13 and 26 data points respectively, were applied to the rectified EMG signal (Figure 1.2), since filtering may affect the onset calculation and as shown by Kadaba et al. (1985) also the repeatability of EMG phasic activity. As the detection threshold has shown to be a major factor influencing onset time detection (Winter, 1984) we tested three different thresholds, namely the mean plus 2, 3 or 4 standard deviations of the raw rectified activity, recorded prior to the tilting. For IEMG calculation the EMG signals were rectified and smoothed using a second order Butterworth filter with a cut-off frequency of 10 Hz. The filtered data were normalised as follows (Arampatzis et al., 2001).

$$EMG_{Nk} = \frac{EMG_{Fk}}{Max_k} \cdot 100$$

EMG_{Nk}: normalised EMG-data from k-muscle
EMG_{Fk}: linear envelope EMG-data from k-muscle
Max_k: maximal amplitude of the smoothed signal from k-muscle of each subject during the first lateral tilt

Then the integrals were calculated from start of the tilt and from each of the six determined onset times to 200 ms after start of the tilt.
The data was split into eight groups resulting from the combination of the three dichotomic categories: stability, expectation and tilt direction. To verify the repeatability of the obtained onset times and integrals we

first calculated the ICCs of all parameters for all three trials from each subject in every condition to asses the linearity of their relationship. Afterwards the Friedman test (a non parametric test for k dependent samples) was applied to check for possible differences (p<0.05) within the set of correlated trials (Yang and Winter, 1983; Kamen and Caldwell, 1996). Finally, to give an idea of the absolute difference between trials, the root mean square differences (RMS) were also calculated.

As an estimator of the sources of variability, the variance due to biovariability and that due to the measurement were estimated as suggested by Brinckmann et al. (2002). The coefficient of variance (CV) was then calculated as the square root of the variance divided by the mean.

$\sigma^2_{bio} = R \cdot \sigma^2_{total}$ $\quad\quad \sigma^2_{bio}$: variance due to biovariability

$\sigma^2_{measurement} = (1-R) \cdot \sigma^2_{total}$ σ^2_{total} : variance due to the measurement

$CV = \dfrac{\sigma}{\bar{x}}$ $\quad\quad \sigma^2_{total}$: variance of the measured values

$\quad\quad\quad\quad\quad\quad\quad\quad R$: Pearson's correlation coefficient

$\quad\quad\quad\quad\quad\quad\quad\quad \bar{x}$: mean of the parameter values

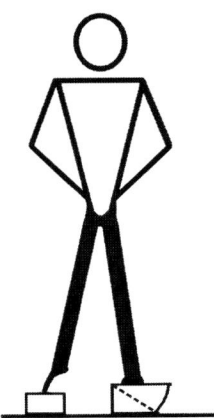

Figure 1.1. Positioning of the subject on the tilt platform. Left foot was full weight bearing having its longitudinal axis parallel to the tilt axis of the plate. The tip of the right foot rested on a block to help maintain balance.

Table 1.2. The onset times were determined using two filters and three thresholds: Mean plus 2, 3 and 4 standard deviations (SD).

Median filter, window width 13 points			Median filter, window width 26 points		
ONSET-1	ONSET-2	ONSET-3	ONSET-4	ONSET-5	ONSET-6
at 2 SD	at 3 SD	at 4 SD	at 2 SD	at 3 SD	at 4 SD

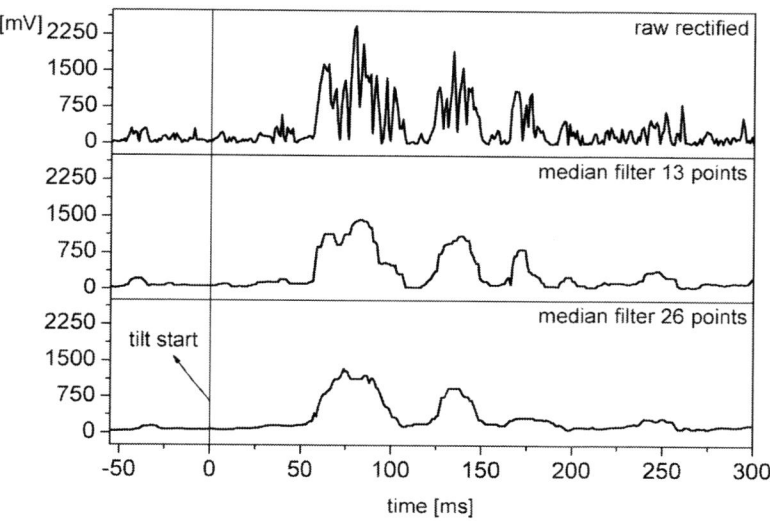

Figure 1.2. Rectified and filtered (13 and 26 points median filter) EMG signal of the m. peroneus longus during a lateral tilt trial

1.3 Results

An ICC above 0.7 was considered to correspond to an acceptable correlation. It is assumed that when no significant differences ($p<0.05$) between correlated trials is found, a higher amount of ICCs above 0.7 corresponds to a better repeatability. As this does not inform about the magnitude of the deviation, the RMS values are also reported. As onset times and integrals have different units, to allow a comparison between these parameters, the RMS values are additionally expressed as a percentage of the corresponding means.

The Friedman test only revealed significant differences ($p<0.05$) between consecutive measures in 2%, 3% and 6% of the cases for onset times (ONSET-1 TO 6), integrals from onset to 200 ms after tilt (INTEGRAL-1 TO 6) and integrals from tilt to 200 ms after (INT.-TOTAL), respectively. Since the results are focusing on repeatability, when citing amounts or percentages of ICCs above certain level, those trials displaying differences ($p<0.05$) between consecutive trials are not included. In order to provide some more information, in table 1.3 the results are split into more levels of correlation.

Onset times vs. integrals: For ONSET-1 TO 6, thirty six percent of all cases have an ICC above 0.7. For INTEGRAL-1 TO 6 and for INT.-TOTAL the corresponding percentages are considerably higher, namely 73% and 81% respectively. The RMS percentages are also higher for the onsets in almost all conditions (Tables 1.4 and 1.5). At all other comparisons done below, the integrals still provide more repeatable results than onset times.

Comparing algorithms: ONSET-1 displays the highest amount of ICCs above 0.7 (44%) and ONSET-3 the lowest one (27%). INTEGRAL-6 has the highest number of ICCs above 0.7 (81%), whereas INTEGRAL-1 has the least (58%).

Comparing trial conditions: Unstable subjects seem to produce more repeatable onset times than stable subjects. No bigger differences are evident when looking at the integrals. Between trial conditions no further systematic differences regarding repeatability can be identified (Tables 1.3 and 1.4).

Table 1.3. Percentage of cases displaying no differences (p<0.05) between correlated trials and having an ICC above given values for the different trial conditions. Data include all muscles and algorithms.

	St-Ux-In		St-Ex-In		St-Ux-Ev		St-Ex-Ev		Un-Ux-In		Un-Ex-In		Un-Ux-Ev		Un-Ex-Ev	
	Ons.	Int.	Ons.	Int.	Ons.	Int.	Ons.	Int.	Ons.	Int.	Ons.	Int.	Ons.	Int.	Ons.	Int.
>0.7	31	67	25	86	39	78	31	75	19	69	50	72	42	89	53	69
>0.8	8	17	8	42	14	72	19	61	17	58	39	50	22	50	39	47
>0.9	0	0	6	8	3	14	6	33	6	8	19	11	14	14	28	19

Stable (St)/Unstable (Un) – Unexpected (Ux)/Expected (Ex) – Inversion (In) /Eversion (Ev)
Ons. = Onset times / Int. = Integrals

Table 1.4. Average root mean square differences (RMS) between trials for the different trial conditions. Absolute values and percentages of the mean. Data include all muscles and algorithms.

	St-Ux-In	St-Ex-In	St-Ux-Ev	St-Ex-Ev	Un-Ux-In	Un-Ex-In	Un-Ux-Ev	Un-Ex-Ev
Onset [ms]	22	29	24	26	20	25	23	20
Int. [%s]	2.40	2.49	3.91	2.76	1.87	3.06	1.91	1.92
Onset [%]	42	79	45	70	43	57	49	62
Int. [%]	32	34	47	35	32	50	40	40

Stable (St)/Unstable (Un) – Unexpected (Ux)/Expected (Ex) – Inversion (In)/Eversion (Ev)
Ons. = Onset times / Int. = Integrals

Comparing muscles: Figure 1.3 should help to better illustrate the repeatability of the parameters regarding the different muscles. The onset times for m. tibialis anterior and m. peroneus longus show quite more high ICC values than those from the other muscles. Interestingly when looking at the integrals, the m. tibialis anterior displays the lowest amount of high ICCs together with m. peroneus brevis and m. gastrocnemius medialis. Table 1.5 presents the absolute and the relative RMS values for the different muscles. Figure 1.3 and table 1.5, besides a lower variability for integrals also indicate that there might be discrepancies between the variability of onset times and integrals.

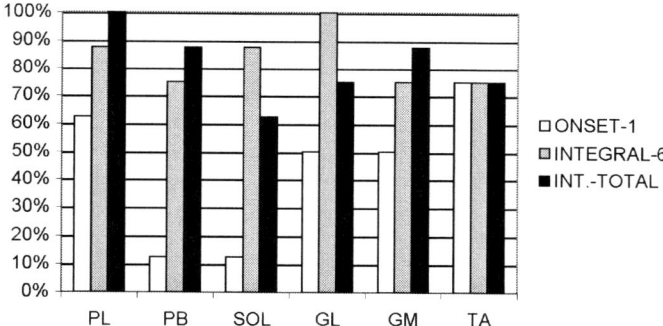

Figure 1.3. Percentage of onset times and Integrals demonstrating an ICC above 0.7 and no differences (p<0.05) between trials for all studied muscles: PL (m. peroneus longus), PB (m. peroneus brevis), SOL (m. soleus), GL (m. gastrocnemius lateralis), GM (m. gastrocnemius medialis) and TA (m. tibialis anterior). Onset-1 and Integral-6 were chosen since they are showing highest number of ICCs above 0.7 for the respective parameter. In addition Int.-total is represented, for it is not dependent on onset times.

Table 1.5. Average root mean square differences (RMS) between trials for the different muscles. Absolute values and percentages of the mean. Data include all groups and algorithms.

	PL	PB	SOL	GL	GM	TA	mean
Onset [ms]	23	25	27	27	30	24	26
Int [%s]	1.74	1.83	2.32	2.85	3.92	5.10	2.96
Onset [%]	52	73	51	48	50	73	58
Int [%]	36	32	32	45	59	64	45

PL (m. peroneus longus), PB (m. peroneus brevis), SOL (m. soleus), GL (m. gastrocnemius lateralis), GM (m. gastrocnemius medialis) and TA (m. tibialis anterior). Onset = Onset times / Int = Integrals

Table 1.6 shows the means and standard deviations of the calculated onset times and the integrals for all muscles and subjects. It can be seen that Onset-1 has the earliest onset detection, followed by Onset-2, 4, 3, 5 and finally Onset-6. The Standard deviations are quite high and similar for all algorithms.

For some subjects, very early onset times together with very low IEMG were observed for some muscles, even when integrating from start of tilt to 200 ms after.

The magnitude of the variability as estimated by the RMS is quite high (Tables 1.4 and 1.5). Also the coefficient of variability due to biovariability is quite high (0.57) and identical for onset times and integrals. That of the measurement was 0.45 and 0.30 for onset times and integrals respectively (Figure 1.4 right).

Table 1.6. Means and standard deviations ( ) of the calculated onset times [ms] and integrals [%s] for all muscles and subjects. Algorithms 1 to 3 correspond to: Median filter window width 13 points; 2, 3 and 4 standard deviations respectively. Onset algorithms 4 to 6 correspond to median filter window width 26 points; 2, 3 and 4 standard deviations respectively. For the integrals the amplitude normalised EMG was integrated from the corresponding onset to 200 ms after tilt start. For Int.-TOTAL the signal was integrated from tilt start to 200 ms after.

Onset-1	Onset-2	Onset-3	Onset-4	Onset-5	Onset-6	
38	45	50	45	52	56	
(29)	(31)	(32)	(32)	(33)	(33)	
Integral-1	Integral-2	Integral-3	Integral-4	Integral-5	Integral-6	Int.-TOTAL
6.62	6.41	6.30	6.45	6.35	6.28	7.15
(3.77)	(3.77)	(3.84)	(3.90)	(4.17)	(4.14)	(4.34)

1.4 Discussion

Concerning the repeatability as estimated by the ICC when no differences ($p<0.05$) between correlated trials is found, in most of the cases the integrals provide quite higher ICC values than onset times (Table 1.3, Figure 1.3). The higher variability of the onset times is also reflected in the higher RMS values expressed as percentage of the mean (Tables 1.4 and 1.5). None of the algorithms used, either for onset time determina-

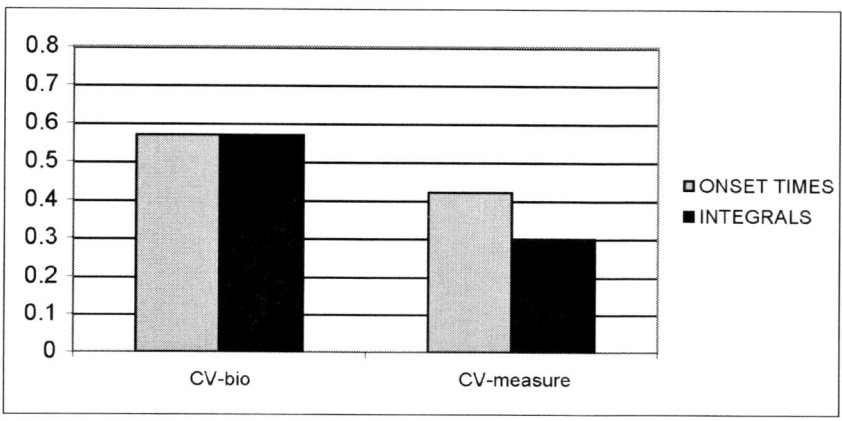

Figure 1.4. Coefficients of variance due to biological variability (CVbio) and due to the measurement (CVmeasure) for all onset time algorithms (Onset-1 to 6) and for all calculated integrals (Integral-1 to 6 and Int.-total)

tion or for the calculation of the integrals, demonstrated a consistently high repeatability for all muscles or trial conditions. This lack in consistency may have several reasons:

a) The interactions between the different conditions might differently affect the reproducibility (e.g. inversion trials producing more repeatable results for m. peroneus longus but less for m. tibialis anterior). So some algorithms might perform better for a given muscle and task combination but not for another. This is supported by our results and to some extent reflected in figure 1.3.

b) The generally high variability of the results also favours a lack in consistency. As shown by the CV, the biological variability seems to play a major role (Figure 1.4).

c) Possibly surface EMG might not be accurate enough for this purpose. One reason might be that EMG is only estimating and not measuring muscle activation. Further, when using EMG only a portion and not the whole muscle is being measured and finally: Biopotentials measured at the skin are very low and despite being measurable, they are very sensitive to artifacts and interferences, which could lead to false onset detection.

The standard deviations in table 1.6 are reflecting the intersubject variability, and therefore do not serve as criterion to judge the accuracy of the different algorithms. However, the intersubject variability is equally described by all algorithms since all of them display similar standard deviations.

Regarding the grouping and the trial conditions the only systematic observation was that unstable subjects seem to have a more constant behaviour regarding the onset times whereas no major differences can be found in the integrals. As the main criterion for subject selection was the subjective feeling of instability, unstable subjects might have been more alert than stable ones, this way achieving a higher reproducibility. Possibly other systematic differences between trial conditions could have been identified if we had taken a bigger sample of subjects and/or amount of repeated measures.

The review of the literature and the presented results indicate that the determination of onset times is critical. Our results show that the integrals during the different intervals considered are quite more repeatable than the onset times and that onset times have only a small effect on the integral itself. Stability studies dealing with EMG focused their attention mainly on reaction times. Some of them find prolonged reaction times in unstable subjects (Konradsen and Ravn, 1990), others do not find any differences (Johnson and Johnson, 1993). For some subjects, very early onset times were observed for some muscles simultaneously having a very low IEMG. This, together with the difficulties inherent to the identification of onset times, might also lead to the controversial conclusions regarding onset times found in the literature and to the questioning of its clinical relevance. Late onset times have been associated to ankle instability (Konradsen and Ravn, 1990). Early but poor activation and later but higher activation could represent two different strategies. When relying only on onset times, it is not possible to distinguish between subjects displaying late onsets and low IEMG and those having the same late onsets but higher IEMG. The first strategy could be hypothesised as risky whereas the second one could represent a safe alternate strategy to early and low activation.

Concluding: Our results demonstrate that relying on only the onset times might be insufficient in many applications. Whenever we are interested in the amount of activity of a certain muscle, we have to use the IEMG or a related parameter. The onset times only provide an instant in time whose determination is critical and which is not necessarily related to the activity occurring afterwards. The IEMG estimates the amount of activity done by the muscle. By setting the integration interval around the expected onset time, useful information relevant to the quality of the onset can be obtained.

Considering the repeatability of both studied parameters and the information provided by them, it is suggested that conclusions drawn about joint stability basing only on the information contained in onset times have to be carefully considered. In many applications the combined use of IEMG and onset times is preferred to the use of onset times alone.

1.5 References

Arampatzis, A.; Schade, F.; Walsh, M.; Brüggemann, G.P. (2001). Influence of leg stiffness and its effect on myodynamic jumping performance. Journal of Electromyography and Kinesiology 11, 355–364

Benesch, S.; Putz, W.; Rosenbaum, D.; Becker, H. (2000). Reliability of peroneal reaction time measurements. Clinical Biomechanics 15, 21–28

Bonato. P.; D'Alessio, T.; Knaflitz, M. (1988). A statistical method for the measurement of muscle activation intervals from surface myoelectric signal during gait. IEEE Transactions on Biomedical Engineering 45, 287–299

Brinckmann, P.; Frobin, W.; Leivseth, G. (2002). B3-Dealing with errors. In: Brinckmann, P.; Frobin, W.; Leivseth, G (Eds), Muskuloskeletal Biomechanics. Georg Thieme Verlag, Stuttgart, pp. 227–229

Di Fabio, R.P. (1987). Reliability of computerized surface electromyography for determining the onset of muscle activity. Physical Therapy 67, 43–48

Duncan, A.; McDonagh, M.J. (2000). Stretch reflex distinguished from pre-programmed muscle activations following landing impacts in man. Journal of Physiology 526, 457–568

Ebig, M.; Lephart, S.M.; Burdett, R.G.; Miller, M.C.; Pincivero, D.M. (1997). The effect of sudden inversion stress on EMG activity of the peroneal and tibialis anterior muscles in the chronically unstable ankle. Journal of Orthopedy, Sports and Physical Therapy 26, 73–77

Gollhofer, A.; Horstmann, G.A.; Schmidtbleicher, D.; Schönthal, D. (1990). Reproducibility of electromyographic patterns in stretch-shortening type contractions. European Journal of Applied Physiology 60, 7–14

Goodwin, P.C.; Koorts, K.; Mack, R.; Mai, S.; Morrissey, M.C.; Hooper, D.M. (1999). Reliability of leg muscle electromyography in vertical jumping. European Journal of Applied Physiology 79, 374–378

Hodges, P.W.; Bui, B.H. (1996). A comparison of computer-based methods for the determination of onset of muscle contraction using electromyography. Electroencefalography & Clinical Neurophysiology 101, 511–519

Johnson, M.B.; Johnson, C.L. (1993). Electromyographic response of peroneal muscles in surgical and nonsurgical injured ankles during sudden inversion. Journal of Orthopedy, Sports and Physical Therapy 18, 497–501

Kadaba, M.P.; Wootten, M.E.; Gainey, J.; Cochran, G.V. (1985). Repeatability of phasic muscle activity: performance of surface and intramuscular wire electrodes in gait analysis. Journal of Orthopedic Research 3, 350–359

Kamen, G.; Caldwell, G.E. (1996). Physiology and interpretation of the electromyogram. Journal of Clinical Neurophysiology 13, 366–384

Konradsen, L.; Ravn, J.B. (1990). Ankle instability caused by prolonged peroneal reaction time. Acta Orthopaedica Scandinavica 61, 388–390

Lynch, S.A.; Eklund, U.; Gottlieb, D.; Renstrom, P.A.; Beynnon, B. (1996). Electromyographic latency changes in the ankle musculature during inversion moments. The American Journal of Sports Medicine 24, 362–369

McKinley, P.; Pedotti, A. (1992). Motor strategies in landing from a jump: the role of skill in task execution. Experimental Brain Research 90, 427–440

Mero, A.; Komi, P.V. (1986). Force-, EMG-, and elasticity velocity relationship at submaximal, maximal and supramaximal running speeds in sprinters. European Journal of Applied Physiology and Occupational Physiology 55, 553–561

Tomberg, C.; Levarlet-Joye, H.; Desmedt, J.E. (1991). Reaction times recording methods: reliability and EMG analysis of patterns of motor commands. Electroencefalography & Clinical Neurophysiology 81, 269–278

Vaes, P.; Van Gheluwe, B.; Duquet, W. (2001). Control of acceleration during sudden ankle supination in people with unstable ankles. Journal of Orthopedy, Sports and Physical Therapy 31, 741–752

Winter, D.A. (1984). Pathologic gait diagnosis with computer-averaged electromyographic profiles. Arch Phys Med Rehabil 65, 393–398

Yang, J.F.; Winter, D.A. (1983). Electromyography reliability in maximal and submaximal isometric contractions. Archives of physical medicine and rehabilitation. 64, 417–420

Zhou, S.; Lawson, D.L.; Morrison, W.E.; Fairweather, I. (1995). Electromechanical delay in isometric muscle contractions evoked by voluntary, reflex and electrical stimulation. European Journal of Applied Physiology 70, 138–145

2 Second Study: Joint stabilising response to expected and unexpected tilts

Study 1 was rather concerned with the methodological issue than on joint stabilisation itself. However we considered that it rose up a relevant matter related to the topic being studied. Therefore it was included in this thesis. The following studies, although also dealing with methodological issues, are more concerned with joint stabilisation processes.

Basing on the results from study one, i.e. high variability of EMG onset times, together with a very discrete information (point in time), the apparent need of different algorithms for different muscles, which is not easy to justify, and the possibility of getting relevant information from EMG amplitude related parameters, we decided not to consider the EMG onset times in the remaining planned studies.

In Study 1 we compared EMG onset times to the EMG integrals. This was done, because the EMG integral is one of the most utilised EMG parameters. This way the study could be of more interest to the research community. However, for the following studies, we preferred to use the root mean square (RMS) of the EMG signal, which also estimates the amount of activation, for several reasons. First, the RMS can be calculated directly from the raw signal, provided it is good enough, and possible error sources introduced by additional filtering or smoothing are avoided. Furthermore, the RMS is independent on the time window width for which it is calculated. Integrated EMG will always increase with increasing window width, so in order to compare the obtained values it is necessary to utilise identical window widths or normalise to duration. In contrast, the RMS provides a mean activity for the whole window width, which can be compared with any other window. The remaining studies are not only concerned with EMG but also with the ground reaction forces and the kinematics of the foot and ankle complex. With this second study we enter the field of joint stabilisation.

The literature review revealed several limitations of the existing studies. The most obvious limitation was the study of discrete parameters without considering other covariates. The other main limitation was, that when kinematics were analysed, the utilised models were too simple to account for the complexity of the foot and ankle behaviour. So most of the studies utilised two-dimensional kinematics and observed only one joint. The next three studies comprise a simultaneous analysis of the three-dimensional kinematics of the foot and ankle joint complex utilising a model including three joints, the muscle activity of six relevant muscles of the lower leg, and the corresponding three-dimensional ground reaction forces.

Joint stabilising response to expected and unexpected tilts

Gaspar Morey-Klapsing
Adamantios Arampatzis
Gert Peter Brüggemann

Institute for Biomechanics and Orthopaedics,
German Sport University Cologne, Cologne, Germany

Accepted for publication in Foot & Ankle Int. on January 26th 2005

Abstract

Background: The results found in the literature regarding functional ankle joint stabilisation are controversial. Possible causes are discussed and a study utilising an alternative approach and its corresponding results are presented.

Methods: The response of 22 subjects to unexpected and expected sudden inversions of the foot were compared. This was also done for two groups of subjects classified according to their self perceived stability. A three-dimensional foot model was utilised to describe ankle and foot motion. Electromyographic signals of six muscles of the lower limb as well as the horizontal ground reaction forces were recorded.

Results: Whereas unexpected and expected trials did not show significant differences (p>0.05) in kinematics, higher activation and horizontal force integrals were found for the unexpected trials. Opposite to that, whereas no differences in electromyographic or ground reaction force parameters were found between stable and unstable subjects, the kinematics revealed higher amplitudes and velocities for the stable group.

Conclusions: The awareness of the instant of tilt enhances stabilisation in that the same motion is achieved with a lower muscle activation. Evidence suggests that this is triggered at supraspinal levels. Higher, rather than earlier activation seems to be decisive in joint stabilisation.

2.1 Introduction

One of the approaches for studying ankle joint stability phenomena is to induce sudden unexpected perturbations during quasi stable tasks as standing, walking or landing from a jump (Caulfield and Garret, 2004; Konradsen et al., 1997; Nieuwenhuijzen et al., 2002; Vaes et al., 2001). Most studies sought factors related to stability by comparing parameters gained from two or more populations grouped by stability, therapy, etc. (Johnson and Johnson, 1993; Vaes et al., 2001). Sudden tilts are frequently utilised in these kind of studies. Main attention has been paid to electromyography (EMG), whereas kinematics have only received secondary attention and have been limited to very simple models using electrogoniometry or tilt plate motion (Isakov et al., 1986; Konradsen and Ravn, 1990; Konradsen et al., 1997; Nieuwenhuijzen et al., 2002; Scheuffelen et al., 1993; Vaes et al., 2001).

Most studies dealing with EMG in a joint stability context, focus on the very early period after tilt and more precisely on the EMG onset times. It is then often assumed, that shorter EMG onset times correspond to a better proprioception and that proprioceptive deficits as determined by delayed onset times would be one of the factors causing joint instability (Konradsen and Ravn, 1990; Löfvenberg et al., 1995). However the results found in the literature regarding onset times in joint stability contexts are controversial (Ebig et al., 1997; Isakov et al., 1986; Johnson and Johnson, 1993; Konradsen and Ravn, 1990). One principal cause of this controversy is probably the multifactorial nature of joint instability and the inherent difficulty of its definition in a quantitative way. This has led to many different criteria for subject selection, which might affect the results. The results can further be affected by the differing experimental set-ups (Lynch et al., 1996): One or two leg weight bearing, initial position, tilt amplitude and direction, foot fixed or not to the plate, etc. Another main issue favouring the controversial results can be the onset time determination itself (Morey et al., 2004). Furthermore, the clinical relevance of onset times in joint stability has not yet been established (Benesch et al., 2000; Konradsen and Ravn, 1990).

There is in general only limited knowledge regarding kinematics in joint stability contexts; this is even less during tilt tests. Some studies analysed two-dimensional kinematics in the sagittal plane (Caulfield and Garret, 2002; Konradsen and Ravn, 1990) or in the frontal one (Scheuffelen et al., 1993; Vaes et al., 2001). Riemann et al. (2003) made a three-dimensional kinematic analysis, but same as most other studies they observed only joints proximal to the ankle and did not consider the different foot structures. The only joint stability study found considering motion between midfoot and hindfoot was that from Konradsen et al. (1997). However they limited their observation to the motion between talus and fifth metatarsal in the frontal plane.

The use of unexpected environmental changes is not new in the literature investigating neuronal reflex phenomena (Duncan and McDonagh, 2000; Dyhre-Poulsen et al., 1984), but in the only study found utilising expected and unexpected perturbations in a joint stability context (Nieuwenhuijzen et al., 2002) the foot kinematics were not considered and the EMG analysis was limited to the latencies.

From all the above, the evidence arises that there is a gap in the literature on how joint stabilisation is achieved. Onset times can hardly describe what muscles do to stabilize a joint, kinematics must be taken into account and furthermore the foot can not be considered as a rigid structure in such a context.

In the present study we analysed foot motion and the corresponding EMG and ground reaction forces (GRF) for the first 500 ms after tilt (300 ms for the kinematics). Assuming that appropriate additional information would enhance joint stabilization, we produced two externally identical situations with different stabilization demands by providing information about the instant of tilt: Expected tilts should allow a better joint stabilization than unexpected ones. The aim of this study was to identify the influence of awareness of the instant of tilt on several kinematic, EMG and GRF parameters by comparing expected and unexpected tilts. Furthermore, two populations grouped by their self perceived foot stability were compared regarding their response to the experimental protocol.

2.2 Methods

Twenty two subjects, all active in sports from recreational to competitive level, were assigned into two groups (n=11) according to their self perceived ankle stability (Stable: female 6, male 5, age 26±3 years, height 177±6 cm, mass 69±9 Kg; Unstable: female 5, male 6, age 24±3 years, height 178±6 cm, mass 72±11 Kg). All subjects gave their informed consent, and the experimental protocol was approved by the ethical committee of our university. The bare left foot was placed on a tilt plate so that its longitudinal axis was parallel to the axis of the plate and 6.5 cm apart. The plate axis was in 15° abduction. All subjects underwent at least 3 unexpected and 3 expected sudden lateral tilts (20°) in random order during one legged stance. The subjects were instructed to bear their whole weight on their left leg, look forwards to a spot on the wall and stand as quiet as possible. The tip of the free leg was allowed to touch the ground to help maintaining balance and reduce EMG activity prior to tilt (Figure 2.1). For the expected trials, a countdown (3, 2, 1, tilt) was performed. At the unexpected tilts the plate was released at any time during or even before the countdown.

Figure 2.1.   Positioning of the subject on the tilt platform. Left foot was full weight bearing having its longitudinal axis parallel to the tilt axis of the plate. The tip of the right foot rested on a block to help maintain balance.

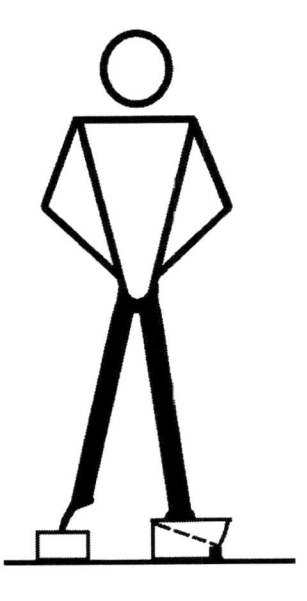

An electrogoniometer (1000 Hz) was aligned with the axis of the plate. Two dampers reduced the impact caused by the plate stop (last 5°). A Kistler force plate (1000 Hz) was situated under the tilt plate. Tilt onset was determined as the instant at which the vertical GRF fell below 90% of its mean value prior to tilt. Foot motion was captured by 4 cameras (2x120 Hz and 2x250 Hz). Bipolar, preamplified (analogue RC-filter 10-500 Hz bandwidth) surface electrodes with an inter-electrode distance of 2 cm were used for EMG collection. The signals from 6 muscles of the lower leg: peroneus longus, peroneus brevis, soleus, lateral gastrocnemius, medial gastrocnemius, and tibialis anterior were sampled at 1000 Hz. EMG and GRF were synchronized by means of a TTL signal which was fed onto both data acquisition boards. Simultaneously four light emitting diodes lighted up, which served to synchronize the cameras with each other and with the remaining systems.

The video data were digitised using the MOTUS 6 software (Peak performance technologies). After obtaining the 3D coordinates from each camera pair, the data were interpolated using quintic splines (Engeln-

Müllges and Reutter, 1991) to achieve a common frequency (1000 Hz). Time zero was defined as the instant of tilt onset. The kinematics of the foot were then obtained by means of a multiple rigid body shank and foot model (Arampatzis et al., 2002 and 2003) (Figure 2.2), which is described at the end of this section. Following parameters were examined: Maximal inversion angle, eversion-inversion amplitude during the first 100 ms, eversion-inversion amplitude between 100 and 300 ms, mean inversion velocity between 20 and 40 ms, and between 10 and 100 ms, and the maximal inversion velocity. The analysed intervals were chosen after visual inspection of the individual and the mean plots of the angular position over time (Figures 2.3 and 2.4).

The root mean square (RMS) of the EMG signal was calculated from the raw signal for five intervals (−70 - −20 ms, 33-100 ms, 100-200 ms, 200-300 ms and 300-500 ms). The EMG data were normalized to the RMS of the EMG during ground contact, while performing defined one legged horizontal jumps onto a 3° laterally inclined surface (the mean from three trials was used). The time around tilt onset was not considered to exclude that possible artefacts caused by the plate release mechanism could influence the results. This information is however present at the mean curves (Figure 2.5) and no noticeable anomalies are seen. Furthermore, latencies shorter than 33 ms are not likely to occur. The shortest latency reported in the literature using sudden tilt tests was 39 ms for the peroneus brevis (Becker et al., 1999).

Figure 2.2. *Lateral, frontal and medial view from a reference measurement used to define the shank-foot model (left) and the graphical representation of the shank-foot model (right) utilised to obtain the kinematic parameters. Note that not all markers used for the model definition in the reference measurement are used for the dynamic tracking of the trials.*

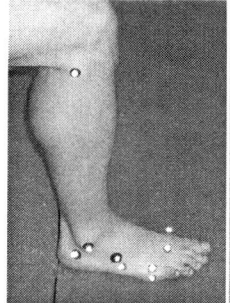

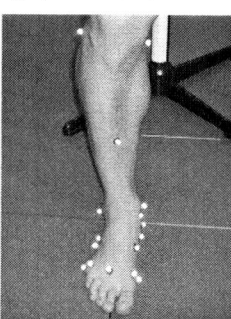

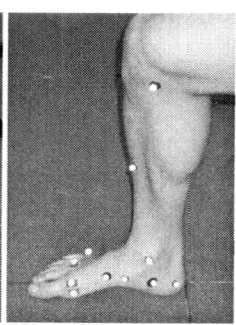

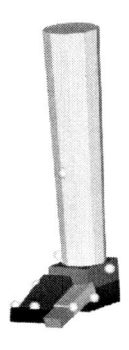

The GRF were normalised to body weight. The absolute values of the positive and negative integrals of the horizontal components (antero-posterior and medio-lateral) were added for five intervals: -200 to –150, 0 to 100, 100 to 200, 200 to 300 and 300 to 500 ms. The first 150 ms before tilt onset were not considered because these values were affected by the plate release mechanism (pulling away a stick). This pulling away was registered by the force plate but is not related to the forces exerted by the subject (Figure 2.6).

The foot and shank model

The lower-leg and the foot were modelled by means of a multi-body system, comprising 4 rigid bodies (Arampatzis et al., 2002 and 2003) (Figure 2.2). For this purpose the simulation software "alaska" (advanced lagrangian solver in kinetic analysis, version 3.0, Chemnitz) was used. The model, which is defined in table 2.1, considers the motion of the hindfoot to the shank (HS), the medial column of the midfoot to the hindfoot (MFH), and the lateral column of the midfoot to the hindfoot (LFH). The three joints of the model do not correspond to real anatomical joints: So the HS motion includes both, the motion at the tibiotalar and the subtalar joints, the MFH motion corresponds to the sum of the motion of all structures included in the medial midfoot to the hindfoot, and the LFH motion corresponds to the sum of the motion of all structures included in the lateral midfoot. However, the model tried to account for the functional anatomy of the foot and allows a more functional examination of the kinematics than simpler models.

Table 2.1. Definition of the segments and joints of the shank-foot model

Segments	Bones	Joints	Connected segments	Degrees of freedom
Shank	Tibia and fibula	Free joint	Space-shank	6 (free joint)
Rearfoot	Talus, Calcaneus	Ankle joint	Shank-rearfoot	3 (ball-socket joint)
Forefoot (medial part)	Os naviculare, three cuneiformi and metatarsals I,II,III.	Medial foot joint	Rearfoot-forefoot (medial part)	3 (ball-socket joint)
Forefoot (lateral part)	Cuboid and metatarsals IV,V	Lateral foot joint	Rearfoot-forefoot (lateral part)	3 (ball-socket joint)

For each joint, two joint coordinate systems attached on each of the connected segments were defined. The joint coordinate systems were defined in a neutral position: Subject seated, knee angle at 90°, tibia to floor 90° (in the sagittal and in the frontal plane), longitudinal axis of the foot contained in the sagittal plane. Seventeen reflective skin mounted markers were attached to the left shank and foot of the subjects (Figure 2.2). Eight markers were fixed on predefined anatomical landmarks to allow the definition of the joint coordinate systems. Nine more markers were placed on not strictly defined anatomical positions but rather on locations where lesser skin movements were expected. The marker locations are listed below. Five markers (1, 2, 4, 7 and 8) were only needed for the model definition and were detached for the dynamic trials. Inversely to the original model (Arampatzis et al., 2002 and 2003), in the present one, marker 3 (most medial point of the tuberositas naviculare) was kept for dynamic tracking, and a marker above the Os naviculare on the instep was not used.

Bony landmarks
1. 1st metatarsal head (most medial point)
2. 5th metatarsal head (most lateral point)
3. Tuberositas naviculare (most medial point)
4. Os Cuboideum (diagonal superior to the basis of the 5th metatarsal)
5. Medial Malleolus (most medial point)
6. Lateral Malleolus (most lateral point)
7. Medial tibial Condyle (most medial point)
8. Fibula head (most lateral point)

Other markers
9. 1st metatarsal head (medial superior)
10. 5th metatarsal head (lateral superior)
11. 2nd and 3rd metatarsal heads (between 2nd & 3rd metatarsal heads)
12. 1st Metatarsus (more proximal)
13. 5th Metatarsus (more proximal)
14. Medial calcaneus (more anterior)
15. Medial calcaneus (more posterior)
16. Lateral calcaneus
17. Fascies tibiae

The foot model calculates the joint kinematics using Bryant angles (Wittenburg, 1977) in following rotation sequence: Eversion-inversion, dorsi-plantar flexion and adduction-abduction. For this paper only the eversion-inversion motion was analysed.

A more detailed description of the model can be found in Arampatzis et al. 2002 and 2003.

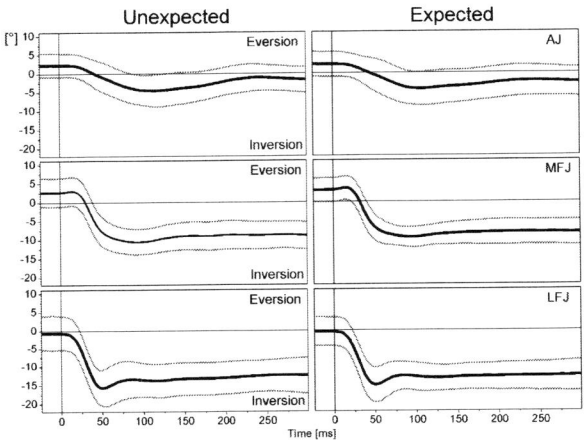

Figure 2.3. Mean ± SD eversion-inversion curves from the unexpected and expected trials. One mean curve per subject and condition was calculated. These mean curves (n=20) were then averaged. AJ: ankle joint, MFJ: medial foot joint, LFJ: lateral foot joint. The vertical line at time zero indicates tilt onset.

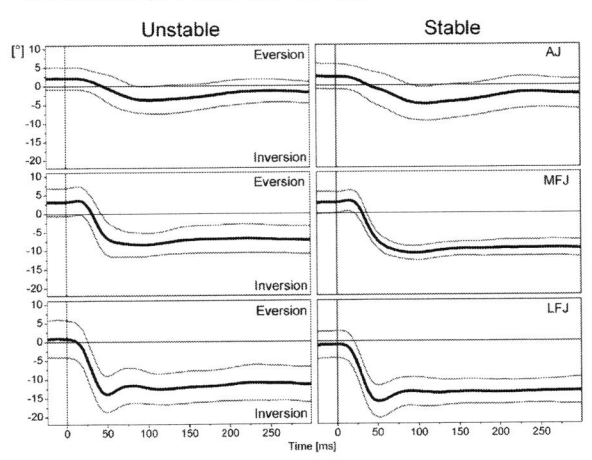

Figure 2.4. Mean ± SD eversion-inversion curves from all trials from unstable and stable subjects. One mean curve per subject and condition was calculated. These mean curves (9 unstable, 11 stable) were then averaged. AJ: ankle joint, MFJ: medial foot joint, LFJ: lateral foot joint. The vertical line at time zero indicates tilt onset.

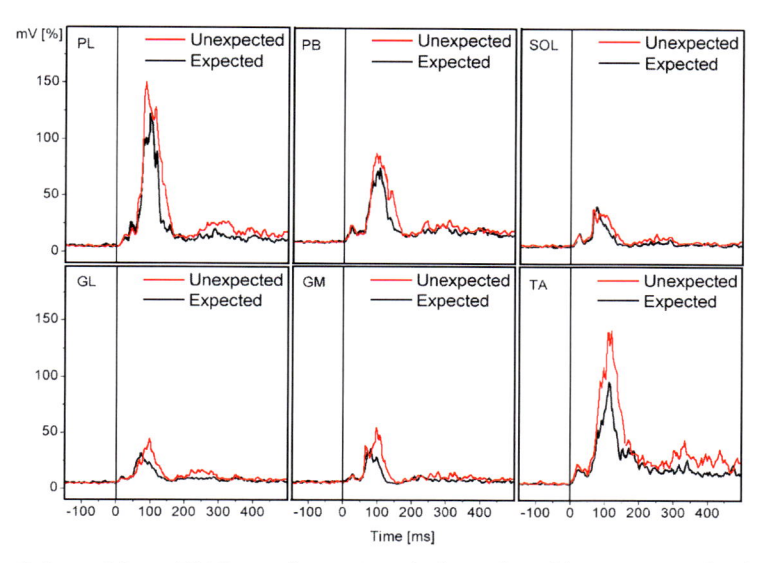

Figure 2.5. Mean EMG envelopes (rectified, median filter 7 points back and forth) from the expected and the unexpected trials. One mean curve per subject and condition was calculated. Then the 22 mean curves were averaged. PL: peroneus longus, PB: peroneus brevis, SOL: soleus, GL: lateral gastrocnemius, GM: medial gastrocnemius, TA: tibialis anterior. The vertical line at time zero indicates tilt onset.

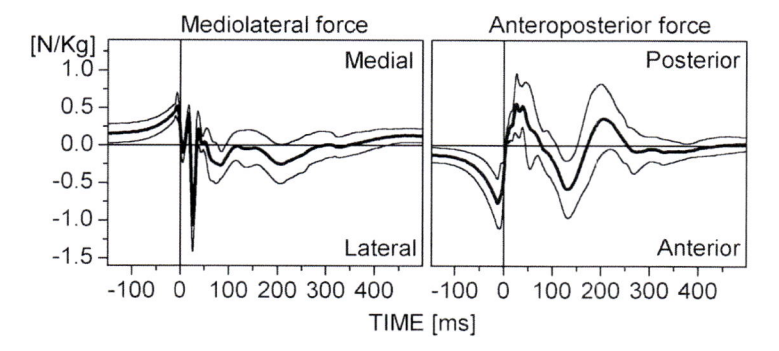

Figure 2.6. Mean curves and the corresponding standard deviations for the horizontal GRF normalised to bodyweight from all subjects during unexpected trials. The vertical line at time zero indicates tilt onset. Note that the force seen before tilt is due to the plate release mechanism, pulling away a stick.

Statistics

All parameters were calculated for every trial. Then the expected and unexpected trials from each subject were averaged, so that one set of parameters from each subject per condition entered the statistic. A paired t-test for dependent samples was utilised to compare expected and unexpected trials. A t-test for independent samples was utilised to compare stable and unstable subjects. In both cases the level of significance was set to $p<0.05$.

2.3 Results

The mean tilt velocity of the plate was 269 ± 33°/s. For the first 15° the velocity was 538 ± 18°/s. For the last 5° (damper) it was 110 ± 23°/s. Total tilt duration was 75 ± 11 ms.

Kinematics

The kinematic parameters did not show any differences ($p>0.05$) between expected and unexpected trials (Table 2.2, Figure 2.3). Whenever significant differences in maximal inversion, motion amplitude, or inversion velocity between the stable and the unstable group were found, the stable group showed higher values (Table 2.3, Figure 2.4). This was seen in two parameters for the HS: amplitude (0 - 100 ms) and mean velocity (20 – 40 ms), and in four parameters for the MFH: maximal inversion (100 – 300 ms), amplitude (0 – 100 and 100 – 300 ms) and mean velocity (10 – 100 ms). No differences ($p>0.05$) were found in any parameter regarding the LFH.

Interestingly, the motion of the hindfoot to the shank was much lower than that of the midfoot to hindfoot (amplitudes 0-100 ms: 6.9 ± 2.5°, 13.3 ± 3.0° and 15.5 ± 3.8°, for HS, MFH, and LFH respectively) (Tables 2.2 and 2.3).

Electromyography

When significant differences ($p<0.05$) in RMS between expected and unexpected trials were found, the values were always higher for the unexpected trials (Table 2.4, Figure 2.5). Comparing expected and unexpected tilts from all subjects together, no muscle showed significant differences in the RMS prior to tilt (-70 – -20 ms). At the interval 33 to 100 ms significant differences (p<0.05) were found at three muscles: peroneus longus, lateral gastrocnemius, and tibialis anterior. All six muscles showed significantly higher values for the unexpected trials at the interval between 100 and 200 ms. Significant differences were also found for the peroneus brevis, soleus and lateral gastrocnemius muscles at the interval between 200 and 300 ms and finally only the tibialis anterior and peroneus longus displayed significant differences in the last interval (300–500 ms). The statistics were also done comparing expected and unexpected trials for only the stable or the unstable group; the results were similar. For simplicity only the comparison for all subjects together is presented. Observing the mean curves (Figure 2.5) expected and unexpected trials display similar timing characteristics. No significant differences were found for any studied interval comparing stable and unstable subjects.

Table 2.2. Mean ± SD of the kinematic parameters from all subjects calculated for the motion of the hindfoot to the shank (HS), the medial midfoot to the hindfoot (MFH), and the lateral midfoot to the hindfoot (LFH) during unexpected (n=20) and expected (n=20) trials. Note that the amplitudes were calculated as the difference between the maximal achieved inversion angle in the corresponding interval and the angular position before tilt.

	HS		MFH		LFH	
	Unex.	Expected	Unex.	Expected	Unex.	Expected
max inversion 0–100 ms [°]	4.2±4.2	4.5±4.3	9.8±4.0	10.1±2.7	14.6±6.1	15.8±4.6
max inversion 100–300 ms [°]	4.5±4.4	4.7±4.4	9.6±4.0	10.0±2.8	13.1±5.7	14.2±3.6
max amplitude 0–100 ms [°]	6.8±2.4	6.7±2.1	13.5±2.6	13.2±2.4	15.6±3.4	15.4±3.7
max amplitude 100–300 ms [°]	7.1±2.7	7.0±2.1	13.5±2.7	13.0±2.2	14.1±2.4	13.8±2.4
mean ang. velocity 20–40 ms [°/s]	83±57	80±62	322±132	353±114	483±174	503±136
mean ang. velocity 10–100 ms [°/s]	71±29	73±24	137±43	144±25	125±46	135±26
max ang. velocity 0–100 ms [°/s]	185±64	191±61	474±183	523±138	590±202	619±172

No significant differences (p>0.05) were found between expected and unexpected tilts.

Table 2.3. Mean ± SD of the kinematic parameters from expected and unexpected trials calculated for the motion of the hindfoot to the shank (HS), the medial midfoot to the hindfoot (MFH), and the lateral midfoot to the hindfoot (LFH) for the stable (n=2x11) and the unstable (n=2x9) group. Note that the amplitudes were calculated as the difference between the maximal achieved inversion angle in the corresponding interval and the angular position before tilt.

HS	MFH		LFH		HS	
	Unstable	Stable	Unstable	Stable	Unstable	Stable
max inversion 0–100 ms [°]	3.6±3.5	4.9±4.8	9.0±3.7	10.7±3.0	14.4±5.6	15.9±5.2
max inversion 100–300 ms [°]	3.9±3.5	5.2±4.9	8.5±3.4	10.9*±3.1	13.0±4.9	14.2±4.6
max amplitude 0–100 ms [°]	6.0±2.0	7.4*±2.3	12.4±2.4	14.0*±2.2	15.2±4.2	15.7±2.9
max amplitude 100–300 ms [°]	6.2±1.8	7.7±2.6	12.1±2.1	14.2*±2.3	13.9±2.7	14.0±2.1
mean ang. velocity 20–40 ms [°/s]	60±64	99*±48	346±142	332±108	489±182	497±133
mean ang. velocity 10–100 ms [°/s]	64±23	79±27	129±36	151*±32	132±43	128±33
max ang. velocity 0–100 ms [°/s]	190±65	188±60	498±179	498±151	608±210	601±169

* Significant differences between unstable and stable $p<0.05$.

Table 2.4. Mean ± SD of the RMS of the normalised EMG signals during several intervals from unexpected (UNEX) (n=19) and expected (EX) (n=19) trials obtained from the peroneus longus (PL), peroneus brevis (PB), soleus (SOL), lateral gastrocnemius (GL), medial gastrocnemius (GM) and tibialis anterior (TA)

	33–100		100–200		200–300		300–500	
	UNEX	EX	UNEX	EX	UNEX	EX	UNEX	EX
PL [%]	99±56	80*±46	86±41	57**±38	43±63	28±26	32±20	23*±18
PB [%]	65±35	65±39	74±43	58*±40	36±21	32*±22	31±17	27±17
SOL [%]	39±16	40±19	27±17	20*±12	24±13	16**±8	16±8	14±7
GL [%]	39±24	34*±20	30±22	24*±24	26±20	18*±18	16±10	15±14
GM [%]	42±31	33±18	29±25	17*±10	19±14	16±11	16±10	13±8
TA [%]	118±141	74*±63	189±197	105*±76	72±88	61±76	77±83	54**±90

* Significant differences between unexpected and expected trials $p<0.05$
** Significant differences between unexpected and expected trials $p<0.001$

Ground reaction forces

The GRF behaved in a similar manner to the EMG. As the GRF in the last 150 ms before tilt were influenced by the plate release mechanism, to control if the ground reaction forces before tilt were differing between conditions, the GRF prior to tilt (-200 – -150 ms) were analysed. No significant differences ($p<0.05$) in the GRF prior to tilt (-200 – -150 ms) nor in the first interval after tilt (0-100 ms) were found between expected and unexpected trials. The last three intervals (100–200, 200–300, 300–500 ms) all showed higher antero-posterior as well as medio-lateral integrals for the unexpected trials (Table 2.5). A plot of the mean curves of the horizontal GRF during unexpected trials together with the corresponding standard deviations can be seen in figure 2.6. No significant differences were found for any studied interval comparing stable and unstable subjects.

Table 2.5. Mean ± SD of the antero-posterior (A–P) and medio-lateral (M–L) integrals of the ground reaction forces measured under the plate during several intervals from unexpected (n=20) and expected (n=20) trials.

Intervals	INTEGRAL A-P FORCES		INTEGRAL M-L FORCES	
	Unexpected	Expected	Unexpected	Expected
−200 to −150 ms [N·ms/Kg]	6.3±4.9	9.5±7.0	8.3±8.3	9.4±6.2
0 to 100 ms [N·ms/Kg]	43.3±18.9	42.1±18.5	32.5±5.9	32.1±5.9
100 to 200 ms [N·ms/Kg]	51.0±25.7	31.4**± 13.3	27.0±15.6	20.7*± 8.7
200 to 300 ms [N·ms/Kg]	37.0±29.1	19.4*± 9.1	28.3±17.8	19.5*± 11.1
300 to 500 ms [N·ms/Kg]	30.7±14.3	22.0*± 7.5	32.0±17.2	21.1*± 10.0

* Significant differences between unexpected and expected trials p<0.05
** Significant differences between unexpected and expected trials p<0.001

2.4 Discussion

In the present study expected and unexpected tilts were utilised to produce different stabilising demands. The aim was to study the influence of awareness of the instant of tilt on several related parameters. In addition the stabilising response of a group with self reported ankle instability was compared to that of a group with no subjective complaints regarding ankle stability.

The main finding is that knowledge of the instant of tilt enhanced the stabilisation process, in that the same foot and ankle motion was achieved with lower EMG activity (no differences prior to tilt). This strongly suggests that the enhanced response to the perturbation is triggered at supraspinal levels. Other studies have drawn similar conclusions with regard to joint stabilisation, pointing up the importance of central patterning and disfavouring the theory of proprioceptive defects as a primary cause of functional instability (Caulfield and Garret, 2002; Gauffin et al., 1988). The higher ground reaction forces during unexpected tilts demonstrate the higher stabilising demands for this condition. No differences prior to plate release could be identified. The ability of muscle activity to maintain foot kinematics at higher demands was also confirmed in a former study analysing landings from different heights onto a gymnastic mat (Arampatzis et al., 2003). The EMG activity of the lower leg muscles increased with increasing falling height but no differences in HS or MFH kinematics were identified. All this suggests that anticipation might play a crucial role in joint stabilisation, especially in unstable subjects. Therefore it could be interesting to focus on this during the rehabilitation process.

The foot complex followed the whole motion imposed by the tilt plate (20°). The HS inverted only about 7°. The remaining motion happened between hindfoot and midfoot. The finding that motion at the HS, i.e. hindfoot to shank, was much lower than that of the midfoot to hindfoot (amplitudes 0–100 ms: 13.3 ± 3.0° and 15.5 ± 3.8°, for MFH and LFH respectively – Tables 2.2 and 2.3) stresses the importance of considering the foot as a mobile, rather than a rigid structure and that focusing only on hindfoot motion might be insufficient in several applications (Arampatzis et al., 2002).

We found the LFH to achieve maximal inversion at 50 ms after tilt and immediately start everting (one degree in 12 ms). The MFH and the HS achieved maximal inversion considerably later (at about 94 and 112 ms respectively) and the following eversion was also slower (one degree in about 43 and 56 ms respectively). Konradsen et al. (1997) found first evidences of active eversion (midfoot to hindfoot measured using an electrogoniometer fixed dorsally above the talonavicular area and the proximal 5th metatarsal) at about 176 ms after tilts of 30° at similar velocities as those from the present study. Their plate rotated 10 degrees more which would take 27 ms. Furthermore, the midfoot was inverted about 26° with regard to the hindfoot, which could make it more difficult to evert; in our case the mean maximal inversion was about 15° for the LFH motion and 9° for the MFH motion. Also the different methods used for motion analysis and the different angle definition may contribute to this difference.

Regarding muscle activation, the biggest differences between both conditions were found for the interval between 100 and 200 ms after tilt. In a similar fashion also the GRF showed differences only after 100 ms post tilt. So, the main influence of awareness on the stabilizing behaviour is not expressed before or immediately after the disturbance but about 100 ms later. This is an important finding if we consider that most of the literature investigating sudden tilts looked only at the EMG onset times (Ebig et al., 1997; Löfvenberg et al., 1995). Furthermore, looking at the mean curves, no apparent differences in the timing pattern can be seen. In contrast, the statistic analysis reveals that the amplitudes of the signal are clearly higher at the unexpected trials, suggesting that in joint stabilisation the EMG amplitude is playing a major role. The fact that the timing patterns are relatively constant may be supported by the findings of Nieuwenhuijzen et al. (2002), who examined the same muscles as the present study whilst walking and stepping onto an unexpectedly collapsing tilt box. They found a similar two burst pattern for the EMG in all muscles. Their reported latencies are very close to the time to peak for the bursts from our data: about 40 ms for the first and near 100 ms for the second burst. Also Isakov et al. (1986) found the peroneal latencies not to be affected by several different tilt axis locations. This could further support the idea of EMG timing patterns not being good discriminators of different stabilising demands, since they do not seem to be very sensitive to changing conditions.

Expected trials display lower mean EMG amplitudes and lower horizontal force integrals. Riemann et al. (2003) stated that the ankle is of primary importance during single-leg stance on firm, foam, and multiaxial surfaces, with proximal joints having an increased role under more challenging conditions. Further, Tropp and Odenrick (1988) found increased horizontal GRF and hip displacement when the body was in disequilibrium while standing on one leg. This suggests, that in our expected trials, whole body stabilization could have been improved by the involvement of other muscle groups at the thigh, hip and trunk, thus reducing the appearing medio-lateral forces and hence the demands on the muscles around the ankle joint as seen by the lower EMG values.

At the imposed tilt (20°) an increased activation of the muscles of the lower leg could account for the unexpectedness in both groups, so that no differences between expected and unexpected trials in foot kinematics were found. The observed foot motion is possibly describing an adaptation to the ground providing a more stable base of support. This can be supported by the fact that the foot remained in its maximal inverted position (only the LFH rotates back about 2.5°) even 300 ms after tilt begin, which is far enough for a voluntary activation to take place. Both groups seem to be able to control foot motion at the imposed tilt (20°). However, higher amplitudes and velocities were found for stable subjects in the HS and the MFH motion when compared to the unstable ones. Possibly the safety limits for stable subjects are wider than those for unstable subjects and at the imposed tilt both groups remain in their corresponding safe zone. It still remains open what would happen at increased stabilisation demands as for example higher tilt amplitudes and or velocities closer to the boundaries of safety. As all subjects were active in sports it could be speculated that the reduced amplitudes represent a protective mechanism in foot and ankle instability. To confirm this, unstable, non active subjects not having had rehabilitation would have to be studied regarding this behaviour. A follow-up during rehabilitation could provide valuable information to identify restoring and compensating strategies. The effectiveness of ankle disk training in improving postural control and the subjective feeling of stability as well as in reducing the incidence of injury has already been demonstrated (Gauffin et al., 1988; Tropp et al., 1985). However, the underlying mechanisms are not well understood. This knowledge could help improving the rehabilitation process.

From all the above some limitations of this study become evident. Models are always a simplification of that what they are representing. Therefore in our case its joints are not representing the anatomical joints of the foot. However this model allows an improved description of the behaviour of the foot and shank with respect to those very simple models utilised in former joint stability studies. Another limitation is that only the shank and foot were analysed, so that possible changes occurring beyond these structures could not be identified. Awareness leads to an improved reactive stabilisation. Therefore supraspinal influences can be assumed. However it remains uncertain what they do. Possible mechanisms could be an improvement of trunk stabilisation, a better coordination of all muscles involved in postural control, or perhaps the main mechanism relies on the enhancement of the reflex action only at the level of the foot and ankle. A last limitation originates from the grouping criterion of the subjects. Subjective feeling of instability, although often utilised, contains no information regarding the aetiology, therefore the conclusions drawn from the comparison between stable and unstable subjects have to be interpreted with care. However this does not affect the results of the main issue of this study which was the influence of awareness of the instant of tilt on foot and ankle stabilisation.

2.5 Conclusions

The main finding is that stable as well as unstable subjects seem to be able to compensate the unexpectedness of the tilts by means of an increased activation of their muscles, resulting into the same motion for unexpected and expected trials. The enhanced stabilisation following expected tilts seems to be triggered at supraspinal level. Another important finding is that EMG amplitude rather than the EMG timing, seems to play the main role in ankle joint stabilisation.

The scarcity of differences between stable and unstable subjects may have several causes: a) sudden tilts of 20° might not be suited to differentiate these groups, b) the subject selection (subjective assessment, all active in sports) might have led to two groups both being able to compensate the imposed tilt, and c) joint stability is a complex multifactorial entity that might be achieved in different ways, and joint instability might be caused by different factors.

2.6 References

Arampatzis, A.; Brüggemann, G.-P.; Morey Klapsing, G.M. (2002). A three-dimensional shank-foot model to determine the foot motion during landings. Medicine and Science in Sports and Exercise 34, 130–138

Arampatzis, A.; Morey Klapsing, G.M.; Brüggemann, G.-P. (2003). The effect of falling height on muscle activity and foot motion during landings. Journal of Electromyography and Kinesiology 13, 533–544

Becker, H.P.; Ebner, S.; Ebner, D.; Benesch, S.; Frossler, H.; Hayes, A.; Gritze, G.; Rosenbaum, D. (1999). 12-year outcome after modified Watson-Jones tenodesis for ankle instability. Clinical Orthopaedics and related research 358, 194–204

Benesch, S.; Putz, W.; Rosenbaum, D.; Becker, H. (2000). Reliability of peroneal reaction time measurements. Clinical Biomechanics 15, 21-28

Caulfield, B.M.; Garrett, M. (2002). Functional instability of the ankle: Differences in patterns of ankle and knee movement prior to and post landing in a single leg jump. International Journal of Sports Medicine 23, 64–68

Duncan, A.; McDonagh, M.J. (2000). Stretch reflex distinguished from pre-programmed muscle activations following landing impacts in man. Journal of Physiology 526, 457-568

Dyhre-Poulsen, P. Mosfeldt Laursen, A. (1984). Programmed electromyographic activity and negative incremental muscle stiffness in monkeys jumping downward. Journal of Physiology 350, 121–136

Ebig, M.; Lephart, S.M.; Burdett, R.G.; Miller, M.C.; Pincivero, D.M. (1997). The effect of sudden inversion stress on EMG activity of the peroneal and tibialis anterior muscles in the chronically unstable ankle. Journal of Orthopedy, Sports and Physical Therapy 26, 73–77

Engeln-Müllges, G.; Reutter, F. (1991). Formelsammlung zur Numerischen Mathematik mit Turbo Pascal-Programmen. Wissenschaftsverlag Mannheim/Wien/Zürich

Gauffin, H.; Tropp, H.; Odenrick, P. (1988). Effect of ankle disk training on postural control in patients with functional instability of the ankle joint. Journal of Sports Medicine 9, 141–144

Isakov, E.; Mizrahi, J.; Solzi, P.; Susak, Z.; Lotem, M. (1986). Response of the peroneal muscles to sudden inversion of the ankle during standing. International Journal of Sports Biomechanics 2, 100–109

Johnson, M.B.; Johnson, C.L. (1993). Electromyographic response of peroneal muscles in surgical and nonsurgical injured ankles during sudden inversion. Journal of Orthopedy, Sports and Physical Therapy 18, 497–501

Konradsen, L.; Ravn, J.B. (1990). Ankle instability caused by prolonged peroneal reaction time. Acta Orthopaedica Scandinavica 61, 388-390

Konradsen, L.; Voigt, M.; Hojsgaard, C. (1997). Ankle inversion injuries. The role of the dynamic defense mechanism. American Journal of Sports Medicine 25, 54–58

Löfvenberg, R.; Kärrholm, J.; Sundelin, G.; Ahlgren, O. (1995). Prolonged reaction time in patients with chronic lateral instability of the ankle. The American Journal of Sports Medicine 23, 414–417

Lynch, S.A.; Eklund, U.; Gottlieb, D.; Renstrom, P.A.; Beynnon, B. (1996). Electromyographic latency changes in the ankle musculature during inversion moments. The American Journal of Sports Medicine 24, 362–369

Morey-Klapsing, G.; Arampatzis, A.; Brüggemann, G.P. (2004). Choosing EMG parameters: comparison of different onset determination algorithms and EMG integrals in a joint stability study. Clinical Biomechanics 19, 196–201

Nieuwenhuijzen, P.H.; Gruneberg, C.; Duysens, J. (2002). Mechanically induced ankle inversion during human walking and jumping. Journal of Neuroscience Methods 112, 133–140

Riemann, B.L.; Myers, J.B.; Lephart, S.M. (2003). Comparison of the ankle, knee, hip, and trunk corrective action shown during single-leg stance on firm, foam, and multiaxial surfaces. Archives of Physical Medicine and Rehabilitation 84, 90–95

Scheuffelen, C.; Gollhofer, A.; Lohrer, H. (1993). Neuartige funktionelle Untersuchungen zum Stabilisierungsverhalten von Sprunggelenksorthesen. Sportverletzung – Sportschaden 7, 30–36

Tropp, H.; Odenrick, P. (1988). Postural control in single-limb stance. Journal of Orthopaedic Research 6, 833–839

Tropp, H.; Askling, J.; Gillquist, J. (1985). Prevention of ankle sprains. American Journal of Sports Medicine 13, 259–262

Vaes, P.; Van Gheluwe, B.; Duquet, W. (2001). Control of acceleration during sudden ankle supination in people with unstable ankles. Journal of Orthopedy, Sports and Physical Therapy 31, 741–752

Wittenburg, J. (1977). Dynamics of systems of rigid bodies. B.G. Teubner Stuttgart

3 Third Study: Joint stabilising response to lateral and medial tilts

In study 2 we analysed the stabilising response to sudden inversions and the influence of awareness on this response. We learned that forefoot motion is much higher and faster than ankle foot motion. So the forefoot motion allows a proper adaptation to the ground, allowing the rearfoot to remain relatively stable. We further confirmed a stabilisation enhancing effect of awareness of the instant of tilt. Only one kind of perturbation was examined. In study 3 we aimed to gain some more knowledge regarding the stabilisation process by means of comparing two different stabilisation demands, identical in magnitude but opposed in direction.

The present study relies on the same methodology as the preceding one. The same kinematic model was used, and similar EMG and GRF parameters were calculated. To our knowledge the existing literature has never examined medial tilts, i.e. sudden eversions. This is surely due to the low clinical incidence of such injuries. However the comparison of lateral and medial tilts might provide relevant information for the understanding of stabilisation processes.

Joint stabilising response to lateral and medial tilts

Gaspar Morey-Klapsing
Adamantios Arampatzis
Gert Peter Brüggemann

Institute for Biomechanics and Orthopaedics,
German Sport University Cologne, Cologne, Germany

In Press (available online)
Clinical Biomechanics (Bristol, Avon)
doi:10.1016/j.clinbiomech.2005.01.008

Abstract

Background: Joint stabilisation processes have been mainly studied comparing groups or joints with different stabilities and mainly focusing on one single parameter. The inherent limitations are discussed and a study where kinematic, kinetic and electromyografic (EMG) parameters gained from sudden tilt tests were measured, is presented.

Methods: The response of 24 subjects to sudden lateral and medial tilts of the foot during one legged stance were compared. A three-dimensional foot model was utilised to describe ankle and foot motion. EMG signals of six muscles of the lower limb as well as the horizontal ground reaction forces were analysed.

Findings: Forefoot to rearfoot motion was faster and greater than ankle motion. In general medial tilts showed lower motion amplitudes and angular velocities than lateral tilts but higher horizontal ground reaction force integrals. The EMG patterns were similar for both conditions. However a specificity of the muscular response could be identified in the EMG amplitudes.

Interpretation: The higher mediolateteral ground reaction forces, together with the reduced kinematic and no general increase in muscular activation in medial tilts suggest, that passive structures seem to be able to counteract destabilising forces and thus reduce the otherwise needed muscular activation.

3.1 Introduction

Functional joint stabilisation, despite being a relatively old issue and having been studied by numerous authors, is not yet well understood. Freeman (1965) stated that "functional instability is usually in first place due to incoordination consequent to deafferentiation". Kleinrensink (1994) started his discussion indicating that "since Cohen and Cohen (1956) proposed the 'arthrokinetik reflex' as a joint stabilising mechanism, several authors accepted ankle stability to be dependent on an intact reflex mechanism". Both theses promoted the idea of joint stability relying on proprioception and motivated most of the subsequent studies in this field.

One typical approach for studying joint stability is to experimentally induce perturbations and observe the stabilising response. In this context, tilt platform tests have been widely utilised and many results regarding muscle onset latencies are available from the literature (Vaes et al., 2001). This is because it has often been assumed, that shorter EMG (electromyography) onset times correspond to a better proprioception and that proprioceptive deficits as determined by delayed onset times would be one of the factors causing joint instability (Konradsen and Ravn, 1990; Löfvenberg et al., 1995). Despite of controversial results, it seems to be generally accepted that there is a link between functional joint instability and prolonged latency times (Konradsen and Ravn, 1990; Löfvenberg et al., 1995). This is further supported by experimental evidences of lowered nerve conduction velocities on stretched nerves or after inversion trauma (Kleinrensink et al., 1994). However there are also several studies that failed to establish the link between latency times and functional joint instability (Isakov et al., 1986; Johnson and Johnson, 1993; Ebig et al., 1997). There are evidences disfavouring the idea of proprioceptive deficits as a primary cause of instability and some studies argue in favour of a main role of central motor programs (Gauffin et al., 1988). Some authors suggested that the main function of reflexes is the updating of motor programs rather than the maintenance of posture in acute situations (Hayes, 1982; Nielsen, 2004).

In a recent review on neural control of movement Nielsen (2004) claims for the need to combine the neurophysiological and the biomechanic/kinematic research traditions to progress in our understanding of motor control. Both traditions have dealt with joint stabilisation. As an example, Bonasera and Nichols (1996) studied the reflex organisation of ankle stabilizers and plantarflexors in decerebrate cats. This study provided experimental evidence on various inhibitory and excitatory neural pathways connecting several muscles around the cat's ankle. However these highly controlled experiments are done in a very artificial context and it remains open to which extent their results can apply to natural motion. Some other studies done on humans have utilised indirect approaches to examine functional neuronal pathways or interneuronal relationships (see Nielsen, 2004). Most studies pertaining to the biomechanic/kinematic tradition have tried to gain insight into joint stabilisation by means of comparisons between sound and affected joints (Karlsson et al., 1992; Vaes et al., 2001) or populations of stable and unstable subjects (Isakov et al., 1986; Konradsen and Ravn, 1990). Both approaches have major drawbacks: The multifactorial nature of functional joint instability makes it difficult to find groups sharing the same aetiology. Thus, even if a factor is identified for a specific group, this would not mean that it should be present in other cases of functional joint instability. Furthermore, there is evidence of injury or training to one side to effect the contralateral one (Gauffin et al., 1988; Kleinrensink et al., 1994). Another deficiency of the biomechanical studies dealing with joint stabilisation, especially of the foot and ankle complex, is that the kinematics have been widely disregarded and only very simple models have been utilised. From a former study (Arampatzis et al., 2003) we learned that we can not predict the behaviour of the whole ankle and foot complex by observing only one joint.

One further point is that most studies on ankle stability using tilt plates examined only sudden inversions. So the observed muscular response has been attributed to the induced inversion. The exclusive observation of lateral tilts does not allow to verify if the observed response is really triggered by the inversion or by other factors common to every joint position perturbation.

From all these, it becomes evident, that there is still need of more research and that the link between the neural part of the sensorimotor system and the mechanical stabilisation process still needs to be enlightened. In the present study rather than identifying factors related to functional instability, it is tried to provide knowledge regarding the stabilisation process itself. So the aim of this study was to examine the influence of two different stabilising demands (lateral and medial tilts) on several related kinematic, kinetic and electromyographic parameters, in order to describe the stabilisation process. Our principal hypotheses were: a. The main adaptation of the foot to the moving plate happens at the midfoot joints rather than at the ankle joint, and b. The primary content of the muscular stabilising response is not triggered by simple stretch reflexes.

3.2 Methods

Twenty four subjects, 12 male and 12 female, all active in sports from recreational to competitive level, participated in this study: Weight: 70.6 (SD 10.3) Kg, height: 177 (SD 6) cm. All subjects gave their informed consent, and the experimental protocol was approved by the intern ethical committee. The bare left foot was full weight bearing and freely resting on a tilt plate. The longitudinal axis of the foot (posterior midpoint of the calcaneus to second metatarsal head) was placed parallel to the axis of rotation of the plate at a distance of 6.5 cm. The plate axis and hence the foot were in 15° abduction. All subjects underwent lateral and medial sudden unexpected tilts (20°) during one legged stance. All trials for one tilt direction were consecutive. After at least 3 successful trials were recorded, the other tilt direction was tested. This was done in random order. The subjects were instructed to bear their whole weight on their left leg, look forwards to a spot on the wall and stand as quiet as possible. The tip of the free leg was allowed to touch the ground to help maintaining balance and reduce EMG activity prior to tilt.

A highly linear potentiometer (10K Ohm, linearity ± 1%, Megatron, Munich, Germany) was aligned with the axis of the plate and provided data describing the plate rotation at a rate of 1000 Hz. Two dampers reduced the impact caused by the plate stop (last 5°). A force plate (Kistler, type: 9881B21, Winterthur, Switzerland) operating at 1000 Hz was situated under the tilt plate. Tilt onset was determined as the instant at which the vertical GRF (ground reaction forces) fell below 90% of its mean value prior to tilt. Foot motion was captured by 4 cameras: 2x120 Hz (60/120 Hz NTSC, Peak Performance Technologies, Inc. Centennial, CO-USA) and 2x250 Hz (one Redlake 250C and one KODAK Motion Corder Analyzer SR-500c, Roper Scientific MASD, SanDiego, CA-USA). Bipolar, preamplified (analogue RC-filter 10-500 Hz bandwidth) surface electrodes (Biovision, Wehrheim, Germany) with an interelectrode distance of 2 cm were used for EMG collection. The signals from 6 muscles of the lower leg: peroneus longus, peroneus brevis, soleus, gastrocnemius lateralis, gastrocnemius medialis, and tibialis anterior were sampled at 1000 Hz. EMG and GRF were synchronized by means of a TTL signal which was fed onto both data acquisition boards. Simultaneously four parallel switched light emitting diodes lighted up. These served to synchronize the cameras with each other and with the remaining systems.

The video data were digitised using the MOTUS 6 software (Peak Performance Technologies, Inc. Centennial, CO-USA). After obtaining the 3D coordinates from each camera pair, the data were interpolated using quintic splines to achieve a common frequency (1000 Hz). Time zero was defined as the instant of tilt onset. The kinematics of the foot were then obtained by means of a multiple rigid body shank and foot model (Arampatzis et al., 2002 and 2003) (Figure 3.1), which is described at the end of this section. Only the eversion-inversion motion was considered for this study. Following kinematic parameters were calculated: Motion amplitudes from 0 to 50 ms, and 50 to 200 ms; mean velocities from 20 to 40 ms (which should approximate the maximal velocity but being less variable) and 10 to 100 ms (representing the mean velocity during the whole tilt), and maximal velocity (Figures 3.2 and 3.5). To allow the comparison between the angular velocities from lateral and medial tilts, the eversion-inversion velocities were calculated as absolute values.

The EMG response is described by the root mean square (RMS) of the raw signals for four intervals (0–50 ms, 50–200 ms, 200–500 ms and 0–200 ms). These intervals fit fairly well to the burst pattern of all studied muscles (Figure 3.3). The EMG data were normalised to the RMS of the EMG during ground contact, while performing defined one legged horizontal jumps onto a 3° laterally inclined surface (the mean from three trials was used). For a better visualisation of the EMG signal, this was rectified and filtered using a 7 point median filter back and forth (Figure 3.3).

The GRF were normalised to body weight. The sum of the absolute values of the positive and negative integrals was calculated for both horizontal force components (anteroposterior and mediolateral) (Figure 3.4) for the same four intervals as the EMG.

All parameters were calculated for every trial. Then the lateral and medial trials from each subject were averaged, so that one set of parameters from each subject per condition entered the statistic. A paired t-test for dependent samples was utilised to compare lateral and medial trials. The level of significance was set to $p<0.05$.

The foot and shank model

The lower-leg and the foot were modelled by means of a multi-body system, comprising 4 rigid bodies (Arampatzis et al., 2002 and 2003) (Figure 3.1). For this purpose the simulation software "alaska" (advanced lagrangian solver in kinetic analysis, version 3.0, Chemnitz, Germany) was used. The model, which is defined below, considers the motion between rearfoot and shank (from now on referred to as ankle joint), the medial column of the forefoot to the rearfoot (from now on referred to as medial foot joint), and the lateral column of the forefoot to the rearfoot (from now on referred to as lateral foot joint). The motion at the ankle joint includes both, the motion at the tibiotalar and the subtalar joints. The motion calculated for the medial foot joint corresponds to the sum of the motion of all structures included in the medial forefoot. In the same manner, the motion of the lateral foot joint corresponds to the motion of all structures included in the lateral forefoot. Due to these simplifications the model does not describe the true motion of the foot bones. However, the model tried to account for the functional anatomy of the foot and allows the examination of the kinematics in a more functional way than simpler models.

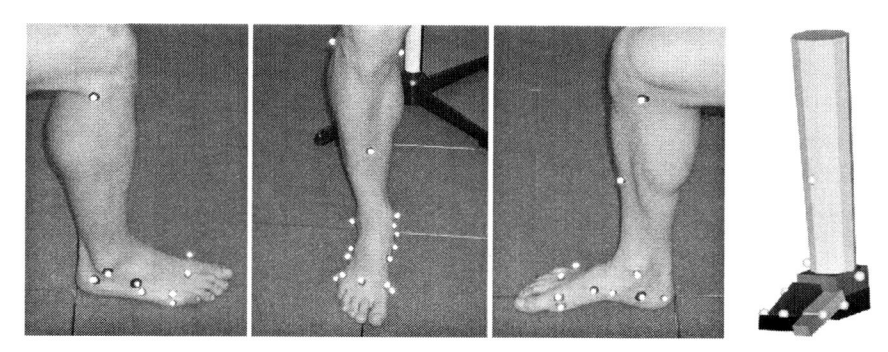

Figure 3.1.   *Lateral, frontal and medial view of the foot and shank with all markers fixed, as placed for the reference measurement. At the right side a view of the model. For this study only four rigid bodies were considered: Shank, rearfoot, medial forefoot and lateral forefoot.*

For each joint, two joint coordinate systems attached on each of the connected segments were defined. The joint coordinate systems were defined in a neutral position: Subject seated, knee angle at 90°, tibia to floor 90° (in the sagittal and in the frontal plane), longitudinal axis of the foot contained in the sagittal plane. Seventeen reflective skin mounted markers were attached to the left shank and foot of the subjects (Table 3.1, Figure 3.1). Eight markers were fixed on predefined anatomical landmarks to allow the definition of the joint coordinate systems. Nine more markers were placed on not strictly defined anatomical positions but rather on locations where lesser skin movements were expected. Five markers (1, 2, 4, 7 and 8) were only needed for the model definition and were detached for the dynamic trials. Inversely to the original model (Arampatzis et al., 2002 and 2003), in the present one, marker 3 (most medial point of the tuberositas naviculare) was kept for dynamic tracking. A marker on the instep above the Os naviculare utilised in the original model was not used. This was done because marker 3 showed to be more stable during movement than the marker on the instep above the Os naviculare.

The kinematics of the ankle, the medial and the lateral foot joints, were defined by the orientation of the most distal joint coordinate system with respect to the more proximal one. Eversion-inversion, dorsi-plantar flexion and adduction-abduction were defined utilising the Bryant angles (a,b,g) describing the rotations about the corresponding axis for each motion. For this paper only the eversion-inversion motion was analysed. A more detailed description of the model can be found in Arampatzis et al. 2002 and 2003.

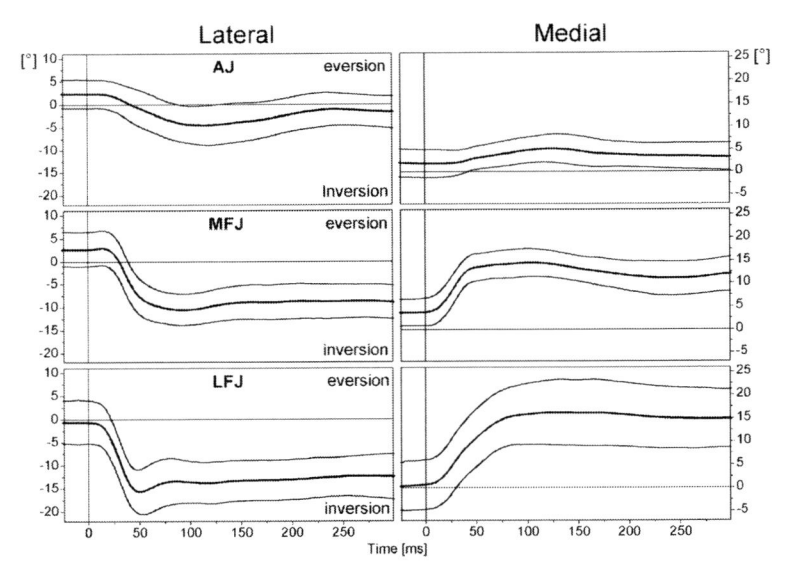

Figure 3.2.   Mean and standard deviation of the eversion–inversion motion for the ankle joint (AJ), the medial forefoot joint (MFJ) and the lateral forefoot joint (LFJ), during lateral and medial tilts (n=20)

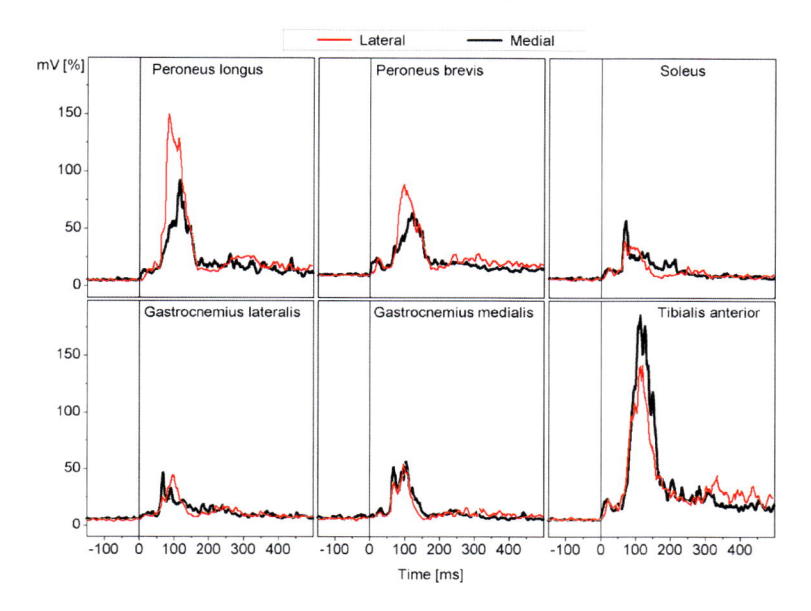

Figure 3.3. Mean curves of the EMG signals from the peroneus longus (PL), peroneus brevis (PB), soleus (SOL), gastrocnemius lateralis (GL), gastrocnemius medialis (GM) and tibialis anterior (TA) for lateral and medial tilts (n=20)

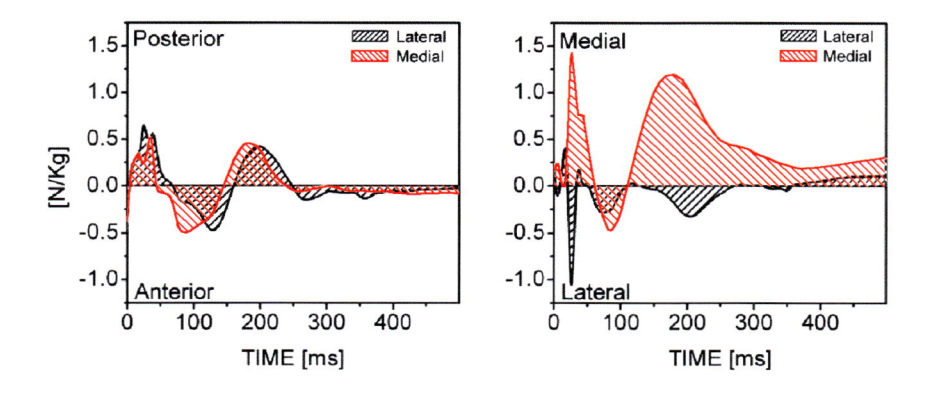

Figure 3.4. Anteroposterior (left) and mediolateral (right) ground reaction forces during lateral and medial tilts (n=24)

Table 3.1. Markers used to define and steer the foot and shank model.

Bony landmarks	Other markers
1. Caput metatarsale I (most medial point)	9. Caput metatarsale I (medial superior)
2. Caput metatarsale V (most lateral point)	10. Caput metatarsale V (lateral superior)
3. Tuberositas naviculare (most medial point)	11. Caput metatarsale II-III (between 2nd & 3rd metatarsal heads)
4. Os Cuboideum (diagonal superior to the basis of the 5th metatarsal)	12. Metatarsus I (more proximal)
5. Malleolus medialis (most medial point)	13. Metatarsus V (more proximal)
6. Malleolus lateralis (most lateral point)	14. Calcaneus medial (more anterior)
7. Condilus medialis tibiae (most medial point)	15. Calcaneus medial (more posterior)
8. Caput fibula (most lateral point)	16. Calcaneus lateral
	17. Fascies tibiae

The bony landmarks are used to define the model, whereas the other markers are only needed to track the motion. See also figure 1.

3.3 Results

Four parameters describing the tilt plate motion were calculated: Mean velocity for the whole tilt (0–20°), mean velocity during the first 15° (undamped), mean velocity during the last 5° (damped), and total tilt duration. All four parameters were significantly different ($p<0.005$) between lateral and medial tilts. Nevertheless the magnitude of the mean differences was small: 5% for total mean velocity and total tilt duration, 1% for the velocity during the 1st 15°, and 7% for the last 5°. The actual values are reported in table 3.2.

Kinematics

As can be seen in figure 3.2, the curves describing ankle joint motion are much smoother than those describing the lateral or the medial foot joint motion. Further, the motion between rearfoot and tibia (Figure 3.5) was much lower than that of the forefoot to rearfoot for both, lateral and medial tilts: Amplitudes 0-50 ms during lateral tilts: 2.90 (SD 1.3°), 9.69 (SD 1.3°) and 14.18 (SD 4.6°), for the ankle joint, the medial foot joint and the lateral foot joint respectively. Amplitudes 0-50 ms during medial tilts: 1.28 (SD 1.0°), 9.89 (SD 1.6°) and 10.04 (SD 2.4°), for the ankle joint, the medial foot joint and the lateral foot joint respectively.

Table 3.2. Means and standard deviations (in brackets) of the tilting velocities and duration for lateral (inversion) and medial (eversion) tilts

	All 20° [deg/s]	1st 15° [deg/s]	Last 5° [deg/s]	Duration [ms]
Lateral tilts	269 (33)	538 (18)	110 (23)	75 (9)
Medial tilts	257* (36)	544* (19)	102* (23)	79 (11)

The last 5° were damped.
* Significant difference between lateral and medial tilts ($p<0.005$)

At the ankle joint all calculated kinematic parameters displayed higher values ($p<0.05$) for lateral tilts than for medial tilts (Figure 3.5). During the medial tilts (eversion) four subjects started slightly inverting the ankle joint and had therefore a negative (inverting) mean tilt velocity between 20 and 40 ms for this joint. As to allow a comparison only the absolute values (no direction information) entered the statistics, this phenomenon is not reflected in the analysis. This, however did not affect the overall results presented here. For the medial foot joint there were no significant differences ($p>0.05$) between both conditions in the amplitudes and only the mean velocity from 10 to 100 ms differed significantly between lateral and medial tilts ($p<0.05$), being 18% higher for the lateral tilts (Figure 3.5). At the lateral foot joint again all calculated kinematic parameters showed significant differences ($p<0.05$) between lateral and medial tilts. For both long intervals (amplitude between 50 and 200 ms and mean velocity between 10 and 100 ms) medial tilts showed higher values (Figure 3.5). This is due to the fact that during lateral tilts, the maximal inversion is reached quite early (mean somewhat before 50 ms) and the lateral forefoot immediately begins everting, whereas at medial tilts, the maximal eversion is reached far later, and almost no recovery (inversion) is seen (Figure 3.2).

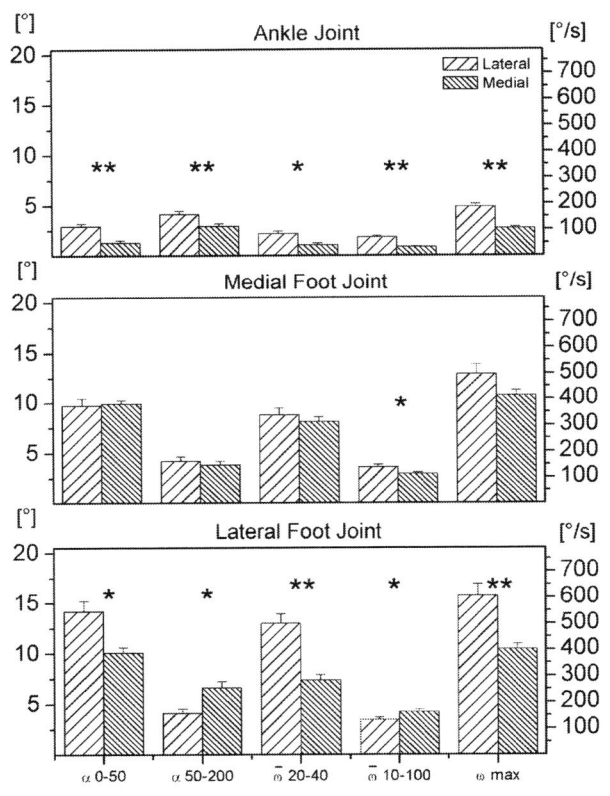

Figure 3.5. Mean and standard error of mean of the kinematic parameters calculated for the ankle joint (AJ), the medial forefoot joint (MFJ) and the lateral forefoot joint (LFJ), during lateral and medial tilts. Parameters: Motion amplitude from start to 50 ms after (α 0–50), motion amplitude between 50 and 200 ms after start (α 50–200), mean velocity between 20 and 40 ms after start ($\bar{\omega}$ 20–40), mean velocity between 10 and 100 ms after start ($\bar{\omega}$ 10–100) and maximal velocity (n=20). Note that the velocities are given as absolute values (no direction). *Significant difference between lateral and medial tilts ($p<0.05$). **Significant difference between lateral and medial tilts ($p<0.001$)

Electromyography

For a better readability the analysed time intervals (0-50 ms, 50-200 ms, 200-500, and 0-200 ms) will be referred to as: early response, main response, late response and early+main response respectively. Observing the mean curves (Figure 3.3) similar shapes of the EMG signals can be seen for both conditions, and differences are only obvious in the amplitudes. For all studied muscles the main burst peaks somewhere between 60 and 120 ms after tilt onset and has a duration of slightly more than 100 ms.

No differences between lateral and medial tilts were found ($p>0.05$) in the early response (Figure 3.6). The main response of both peroneal muscles showed higher values during lateral tilts ($p<0.001$ for PL and $p<0.05$

EMG RMS

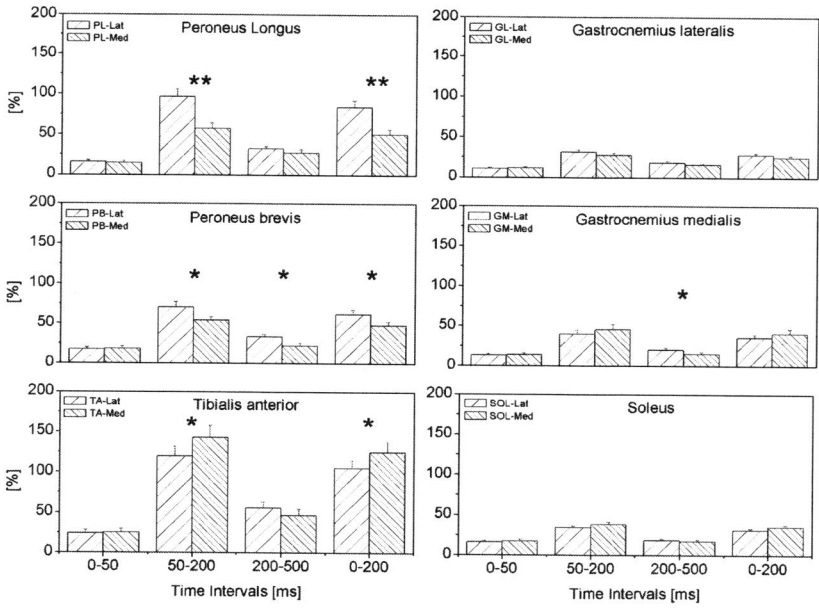

Figure 3.6. Root mean square values and the corresponding standard errors of the EMG signal from peroneus longus (PL), peroneus brevis (PB), soleus (SOL), gastrocnemius lateralis (GL), gastrocnemius medialis (GM) and tibialis anterior (TA) for several time intervals during lateral and medial tilts (n=20). *Significant difference between lateral and medial tilts ($p<0.05$). **Significant difference between lateral and medial tilts ($p<0.001$)

for PB). Oppositely the tibialis anterior showed a higher main response during medial tilts (p<0.05). No differences in the main response between lateral and medial tilts could be found for the muscles of the triceps surae (p>0.05). In the late period the only differences were for the mm. peroneus brevis and gastrocnemius medialis, who showed higher activity at the lateral trials (p<0.05). For the early+main response the results were the same as for the main response (Figure 3.6).

Ground reaction forces

The same nomenclature as utilised for the EMG intervals is used to refer to the GRF integration intervals. In general the anteroposterior forces behaved in a similar manner for both tilt conditions. The curves approximate one and a half sinusoidal cycles, starting with forces in the posterior direction (Figure 3.4). However, the early response showed somewhat higher values (p<0.001) for the lateral trials (Figure 3.7). The mediolateral force plots, obviously reflect the tilt direction in that the medial component is dominant for medial tilts and the lateral one during lateral tilts (Figure 3.4). Further, all calculated mediolateral force integrals were higher (p<0.001) for the medial tilts (Figure 3.7).

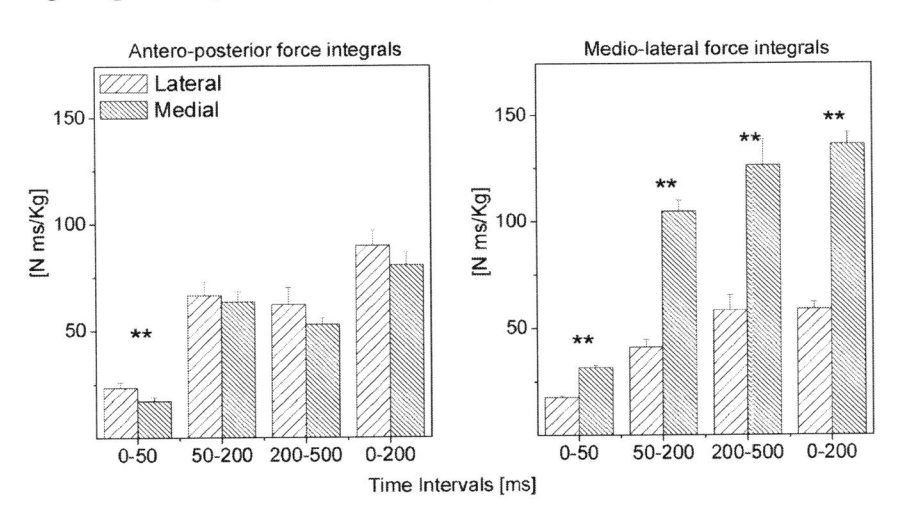

Figure 3.7. Integrals of the mediolateral and the anteroposterior force integrals for several time integrals (n=24)

3.4 Discussion

The present study aimed to examine the influence of two different stabilising demands (lateral and medial tilts) on several related kinematic, kinetic and electromyographic parameters, in order to describe the stabilisation process. For both conditions tilt duration was slightly below 80 ms. The ankle joint rotated clearly slower and to a lesser amount than the plate. The forefoot to rearfoot motion achieved similar velocities than the plate and after the end of tilt plate rotation there were only minor increases in joint motion amplitude. The EMG burst appears when maximal amplitude is almost reached and the velocity is already lowered to some extent (compare figures 3.2 and 3.3). The GRFs are still quite high even after the EMG signals are almost extinguished (compare figures 3.3 and 3.4).

Despite care was taken in placing the foot onto the tilt plate with its longitudinal axis 6.5 cm apart from the tilt axis for both conditions, the tilt velocities differed between lateral and medial trials (Table 3.2). The higher velocities for medial tilts during the initial undamped 15° could be caused by the subjects having their point of force application under the foot slightly medial to its longitudinal axis (posterior midpoint of the calcaneus to second metatarsal head). This would lead to a longer moment arm for the medial tilts and a shorter one for the lateral ones. So, assuming identical forces, the moment around the axis of the plate would be higher for medial tilts and consequently also the tilt velocities. The lower velocity for medial tilts during the last 5° of damped motion are probably representing a functional phenomenon. However, the differences despite being significant ($p<0.05$) were low (mean total tilt duration only 4 ms longer for medial tilts). Therefore no substantial effect on the presented results is expected.

One main finding was that the motion amplitudes and the corresponding velocities are considerably higher for the joints between fore and rearfoot than between rearfoot and tibia. This was up to twice as high for lateral tilts and more than three times higher for the medial tilts (Figures 3.2 and 3.5). Similar findings were reported by Arampatzis et al. (2002), where the same foot model was utilised to study landings on gymnastic mats with different stiffness. They found the maximal eversion angles at the medial foot joint and the lateral foot joint to be approximately two and three times that of the ankle joint. Further Arampatzis et al. (2002) reported, that the motion at the AJ in contrast to that at the other two joints, was not affected by mat stiffness. This reinforces the importance of considering the foot as a mobile rather than a rigid structure, since the same behaviour in one joint does not necessarily serve to predict that of the others.

Hypothesis a. was confirmed. In the present study the joints between forefoot and rearfoot followed most of the motion of the plate in a relatively unconstrained way for the first 15° of tilt (about 27 ms). As most of the motion occurred in these joints, there was no need for the ankle to follow the whole motion of the tilt plate. For lateral tilts the sum of the motion between forefoot and rearfoot and between rearfoot and shank corresponds fairly well to the 20° of plate motion. However the joints rotated back to some extent and did not remain in this position. For the medial tilts this sum was somewhat lower, indicating that the foot complex did not completely adapt to the plate motion. Despite ranges of motion of 20° in both directions have been described even for the ankle joint alone, the flexibility (°/Nm) is significantly lower for eversion (Siegler et al., 1994). This could explain the fact that the medial tilts led to higher horizontal force integrals (about twice as high $p<0.001$) than the lateral tilts without leading to higher angular excursions or velocities (in fact these were lower) nor to a generally increased muscular activation.

Another important finding arising from the comparison of lateral and medial tilts was that the specificity of the muscular response i.e. the higher activation of the peroneal muscles during lateral tilts (inversion) and the higher activation of the tibialis anterior (which has an inverting component) during medial tilts (eversion), is rather expressed in the level of activation than in timing. There were almost no differences in the activation of the triceps surae muscles.

The lower activity seen for the peroneus brevis and the gastrocnemius medialis in the late response during medial tilts, could be an indicator for an easier stabilisation in this condition. A possible explanation would be that the higher motion restriction provided by the passive structures during medial tilts relieves the neuromuscular system, facilitating the stabilisation task by reducing the degrees of freedom to be controlled.

Finally, the fact that the peroneal muscles show very similar activation profiles for both conditions, despite of not being stretched during the medial tilts, strongly suggests that there is only a partial contribution of stretch reflexes to the overall response. This same reasoning would apply to the behaviour of the tibialis anterior which is stretched during medial but not lateral tilts. So hypothesis b. is confirmed. This partial contribution of the stretched structures to the activation could account for the specificity of the response (higher amplitudes in those muscles counteracting the induced motion). Our results are in agreement with those of Myers et al. (2003), who found that anaesthesia of the periferal afferents to the ankle ligaments protecting against inversion, did not effect muscle reflex latencies but EMG amplitudes. However it should not be neglected, that the subjects knew they were about to tilt and were aware of the direction of the tilt. It is therefore possible that also central feedforward mechanisms contributed to the general but also the specific muscular response.

3.5 Conclusions

During stabilisation following perturbation, forces are generated (kinetics and muscle activity) to counteract the perturbation and restore or achieve a new stable position (kinematics and kinetics). Therefore when trying to understand such processes it is important to take into account at least these factors: kinematics, kinetics and muscle activity. Concerning foot and ankle stabilisation, the foot should not be considered as a rigid structure. Too simple models could produce misleading results, as they can not describe the behaviour of the whole foot. Basing on the collected EMG data it can be argued that studying functional joint stabilisation only by focusing on agonistic stretch reflexes is too limited to explain the functioning of this system and its pathology. Future studies should consider the whole EMG signal rather than only latency times. Finally the possible influence from central processes as well as from factors others than simple stretch reflexes should not be neglected when planning any experimental design in this area.

We studied the response to sudden ankle position perturbations in the frontal plane. Forces were generated to counteract the perturbation. For medial tilts the passive constraints seem to account for this forces to a higher extent than for lateral tilts. It is suggested that the narrower constraints to eversion relief the neuromuscular system and facilitate the stabilisation process.

3.6 References

Arampatzis, A.; Brüggemann, G.-P.; Morey Klapsing, G.M. (2002). A three-dimensional shank-foot model to determine the foot motion during landings. Medicine and Science in Sports and Exercise 34, 130–138

Arampatzis, A.; Morey Klapsing, G.M.; Brüggemann, G.-P. (2003). The effect of falling height on muscle activity and foot motion during landings. Journal of Electromyography and Kinesiology 13, 533–544

Bonasera, S.J.; Nichols, T.R. (1996). Mechanical actions of heterogenic reflexes among ankle stabilizers and their interactions with plantarflexors of the cat hindlimb. Journal of Neurophysiology 75, 2050–2070

Cohen, L.A.; Cohen, M.L. (1956). Arthrokinetic reflex of the knee. American Journal of Physiology. 184, 433–437

Ebig, M.; Lephart, S.M.; Burdett, R.G.; Miller, M.C.; Pincivero, D.M. (1997). The effect of sudden inversion stress on EMG activity of the peroneal and tibialis anterior muscles in the chronically unstable ankle. Journal of Orthopedy, Sports and Physical Therapy 26, 73–77

Freeman, M.A.; Dean, M.R.; Hanham, I.W. (1965). The etiology and prevention of functional instability of the foot. Journal of Bone and Joint Surgery 47, 678–685

Gauffin, H.; Tropp, H.; Odenrick, P. (1988). Effect of ankle disk training on postural control in patients with functional instability of the ankle joint. Journal of Sports Medicine 9, 141–144

Hayes, K.C. (1982). Biomechanics of postural control. Exercise and Sport Sciences Reviews 10, 363–391

Isakov, E.; Mizrahi, J.; Solzi, P.; Susak, Z.; Lotem, M. (1986). Response of the peroneal muscles to sudden inversion of the ankle during standing. International Journal of Sports Biomechanics 2, 100–109

Johnson, M.B.; Johnson, C.L. (1993). Electromyographic response of peroneal muscles in surgical and nonsurgical injured ankles during sudden inversion. Journal of Orthopedy, Sports and Physical Therapy 18, 497–501

Karlsson, J.; Peterson L.; Andreasson, G.; Hogfors, C. (1992). The unstable ankle, A combined EMG and Biomechanical Modeling Study. International Journal of Sports Biomechanics 8, 129–144

Kleinrensink, G.J.; Stoeckart, R.; Meulstee, J.; Kaulesar Sukul, D.M.; Vleeming, A.; Snijders, C.J.; van Noort, A. (1994). Lowered motor conduction velocity of the peroneal nerve after inversion trauma. Medicine and Science in Sports and Exercise 26, 877–883

Konradsen, L.; Ravn, J.B. (1990). Ankle instability caused by prolonged peroneal reaction time. Acta Orthopaedica Scandinavica 61, 388–390

Löfvenberg, R.; Kärrholm, J.; Sundelin, G.; Ahlgren, O. (1995). Prolonged reaction time in patients with chronic lateral instability of the ankle. The American Journal of Sports Medicine 23, 414–417

Myers, J.B.; Riemann, B.L.; Hwang, J.H.; Fu, F.H.; Lephart, S.M. (2003). Effect of peripheral afferent alteration of the lateral ankle ligaments on dynamic stability. The American Journal of Sports Medicine 31, 498–506

Nielsen, J.B. (2004). Sensorimotor integration at spinal level as a basis for muscle coordination during voluntary movement in humans. Journal of Applied Physiology 96, 1961–1967

Siegler, S.; Wang, D.; Plasha, E.; Berman, T. (1994). Technique for in vivo measurement of the three-dimensional kinematics and laxity characteristics of the ankle joint complex. Journal of orthopaedic research 12, 421–431

Vaes, P.; Van Gheluwe, B.; Duquet, W. (2001). Control of acceleration during sudden ankle supination in people with unstable ankles. Journal of Orthopedy, Sports and Physical Therapy 31, 741–752

4 Fourth Study: Foot and ankle stabilisation during drop landing: A kinematic, kinetic and electromyographic study

The three previous studies were based on sudden tilts whilst standing. Such a setup allows to attain relatively high controlled experimental conditions: Initial foot position is nearly the same for all trials and subjects, EMG prior to tilt is minimised and monitorised prior to releasing the plate, GRF are controlled. Consequently also the perturbation is very similar among trials and subjects. However the obvious advantages of controlled experimental conditions have inherent drawbacks. So the studied situation is a fairly artificial one. In daily life or sports, most of the sudden inversions occur at the instant of loading the foot, and not when the foot is already loaded. Controlled landings provide a suited model to study stabilisation processes. Landings challenge the joint stabilising system, since the perturbation imposed by the collision with the ground is quite fast and of considerable magnitude. As landings allow more degrees of freedom than tilts from a defined standing position, in addition to the eversion-inversion motion we examined the dorsiflexion-plantarflexion and the adduction-abduction motions. Furthermore, as an adequate preparation can be crucial for a successful landing, special interest was paid to the period prior to touchdown.

FOOT AND ANKLE STABILISATION DURING DROP LANDING: A KINEMATIC, KINETIC AND ELECTROMYOGRAPHIC STUDY

Gaspar Morey-Klapsing
Adamantios Arampatzis
Gert Peter Brüggemann

Institute for Biomechanics and Orthopaedics,
German Sport University Cologne, Cologne, Germany

Submitted for publication on March 3rd 2005

Abstract

Several studies have dealt with joint stabilisation processes. Whereas many involved mechanisms have been addressed, most studies focused only on discrete parameters. Recently the need of more comprehensive approaches has become evident. In this study, the response of 24 subjects during one legged landings onto three surfaces, a level one and two surfaces inclined 3° either laterally or medially, were compared. A three-dimensional foot model was utilised to describe ankle and foot motion. Electromyographic (EMG) signals from six muscles of the lower limb as well as the ground reaction forces (GRF) were analysed. The results revealed surface specific responses even prior to touchdown (TD) in the kinematics and the EMG (e.g. higher lateral forefoot inversion and peroneal activity for the laterally inclined surface). The forefoot joints had a more specific response than the ankle joint, especially in eversion-inversion. Similarly the peroneal muscles were more sensitive to surface inclination than the triceps surae mucles. The medially inclined surface led to lower mediolateral GRF near TD, and to a lower vertical force maximum than the laterally inclined surface. Early post-TD responses can be explained by self-stabilizing mechanisms of the musculoskeletal system which are not related to any feedback arising from the collision with the surface. We conclude, that changes in frontal plane surface inclination produce different central motor commands, especially in the frontal plane of motion, possibly aimed to enhance the self-stabilising potential of the whole system. 3° medial inclination seem to provide certain damping and relief the neuromuscular system.

4.1 Introduction

Landings are a convenient model for studying motor control strategies counteracting the external mechanical loads at impact (Duncan and McDonagh, 2000; Pelland and McKinley, 2004). In contrast to a pure feedback control, which is limited to relatively slow adaptations because of the latencies in information flow, feedforward control might provide solutions right in time. Therefore such mechanisms are especially important when the imposed perturbations are fast, as it is the case of foot and ankle stabilisation during landing. The control of landing tasks is an important issue by itself. Landings from moderate heights (~40 cm) are relatively common in daily life. The ground onto which the landing is performed, is not always level. Therefore our neuromuscular system has to be able to adapt to different surface conditions.

Despite a considerable amount of studies done on landings have produced many interesting results contributing to our understanding of the landing process, this issue is not yet thoroughly understood (Santello, 2005). One important but poorly enlightened question that might play a crucial role in the joint stabilisation process after landings is: How is stabilisation achieved during the early phase (first 40–50 ms) after touchdown (TD), where the ground reaction forces (Caulfield and Garret, 2004) as well as the motion of the foot structures (Arampatzis et al., 2002) are highest, and no significant reflex activity can be expected (Dyhre-Poulsen et al., 1991; Grüneberg et al., 2003; Duncan and McDonagh, 2000)? Moritz and Farley (2004) showed that during hopping, passive mechanisms alter leg stiffness in response to surface compliance before changes in electromyography (EMG) are observed, and that anticipative adjustments in muscular activity and kinematics to the surface characteristics were done prior to TD. These results are supported by Wagner and Blickhan (2003) who found particular anatomical and physiological characteristics of the knee joint and its associated muscles to improve its self-stabilizing potential.

Most studies dealing with landings did not focus on the above question. Following, some of the knowledge gained on the landing process will be briefly exposed: Landing technique is highly variable among subjects (Dufek and Bates, 1990; Caster and Bates, 1995). Changes in landing technique might affect the ground reaction forces (GRF) (Arampatzis et al., 2002), and also leg accelerations and Achilles tendon forces (Self and Paine, 2001). Whereas unskilled subjects choose a default technique, skilled ones are able to change their behaviour to adapt to changes in surface compliance (McKinley and Pedotti, 1992). During landings patients with functional ankle instability and healthy controls show differences in sagittal kinematics of the ankle and knee (Caulfield and Garret, 2002) and in the GRF (Caulfield and Garret, 2004).

Considerable changes in falling height, 0.2 to 1 m (Santello and McDonagh, 1998) and 1 to 2 m (Arampatzis et al., 2003) do not affect the kinematics of the ankle joint, but lead to increased EMG activity even prior to TD. Falling height can also influence the forefoot kinematics (Arampatzis et al., 2003).

Slight changes in surface compliance have no significant effect on shock attenuation or sagittal ankle kinematics (Gross and Nelson, 1988). The same applies to the maximal GRF and to the three-dimensional ankle kinematics, but not to the motion between forefoot and rearfoot which was higher onto a more compliant mat (Arampatzis et al., 2002).

Landings onto an inverting surface have lower amplitude short latency reflexes, but higher amplitude long latency reflexes as landings onto a rigid level surface (Grüneberg et al., 2003). When landing onto inclined surfaces, allowing the forefoot to adapt to the ground (foot torsion) considerably reduces the frontal plane motion between the rearfoot and the leg (Stacoff et al., 1990).

Several studies have focused mainly on the EMG activity of landings. A study on the origin of prelanding EMG showed that its modulation may rely on impact force estimation and depend on the availability of sensory modalities (Thompson and McKinley, 1995). Other studies suggest that sensory feedback might play only a minor role in landing control once the task is known and a motor strategy has been developed by means of some practice trials (Dyhre-Poulsen and Mosfeldt Laursen, 1984; Liebermann and Hoffman, 2005). Whereas the importance of an adequate preactivation of the muscles in the control of a subsequent landing is generally accepted, there has been some discrepancy regarding the origin and importance of the activity observed after touchdown (TD) (see Dyhre-Poulsen and Mosfeldt Laursen, 1984; Duncan McDonagh, 2000; Grüneberg et al., 2003).

Approaches based on discrete mechanical or neural viewpoints limit their explaining potential due to the interdependence of most involved factors. Ignoring one factor often hinders the interpretation of the findings (Caster and Bates, 1995; Nielsen, 2004). So, those studies focusing only on EMG (Grüneberg et al., 2003) or GRF (Caulfield and Garret, 2004) or kinematics (Caulfield and Garret, 2002) may observe interesting phenomena, but may have to rely on assumptions in their explanations, since the information regarding the other involved parameters is missing and can at best only be inferred. Some studies delivered more consistent knowledge regarding the mechanics and the motor control of landings by means of combining kinematics, kinetics and electromyography (McKinley and Pedotti, 1992; Santello and McDonagh, 1998). However the complexity of the ankle-foot system has been widely disregarded and too simple models observing only two-dimensional kinematics or only ankle joint motion might be insufficient when dealing with foot and ankle stabilisation. Moritz and Farley (2004) have shown anticipative adjustments in knee angle according to expected surface stiffness and stressed the role of passive self-stabilising mechanisms relying on segment orientation. To study such mechanisms at the foot and ankle complex, which is the structure nearest to the ground and most closely interacting with it, appropriate models are needed. Previous studies have shown that in many cases the foot can not be considered as a rigid structure (Stacoff et al., 2000; Arampatzis et al., 2002 and 2003). Exemplarily some studies failed to detect any changes in sagittal (Gross and Nelson, 1988) and even three-dimensional (Arampatzis et al., 2002) ankle joint kinematics during landings onto surfaces with different compliance. This latter study however, detected differences in the kinematics between forefoot and rearfoot. Such results stress the need of utilising more complex models of the foot and ankle complex including three-dimensional kinematics and not considering the foot as a rigid, but a mobile structure, i.e. dividing it into functional segments. This is especially true when the aim is to observe reactions to ground unevenness (e.g. destabilisation in the frontal plane) (Stacoff et al., 2000). Feedforward adjustments in EMG and sagittal kinematics to landings have been previously reported (McKinley and Pedotti, 1992; Santello and McDonagh, 1998; Arampatzis et al., 2003; Moritz and Farley, 2004). However, up to now no evidence of feedforward control of frontal plane motion has been reported.

In the present study changes in frontal plane surface inclination (laterally and medially inclined) should provoke stabilising responses triggered by different perturbations, identical in magnitude but opposite in direction. We hypothesised that small changes in frontal plane inclination of the landing surface will lead to different functional adjustments in EMG and in the kinematics prior to TD. Furthermore, by means of the simultaneous analysis of its three-dimensional kinematics, EMG signals and ground reaction forces, we aimed to provide a better understanding on how stabilisation is achieved.

4.2 Methods

The present study was approved by the internal ethical committee. All subjects, 12 male and 12 female, aged between 20 and 33 years, all active in sports from recreational to competitive level gave their informed consent to participate in this study. The subjects had to perform one legged drop landings from a 40 cm high box onto three different surfaces situated directly in front of the edge of the box: A level one and two surfaces inclined 3 degrees either laterally or medially (Figure 4.1). The drop was initiated by forwarding the right foot and pushing off from the box with the left one. The subjects were instructed to land on their left foot and stabilise their body as soon as possible. The hands were held on the hips. All subjects had to perform at least three successful trials per condition. A trial was successful when: All measuring systems recorded the corresponding data, the landing was stabilised without touching the ground with the right foot, and there was no hop, i.e. loss of ground contact with the foot after TD. During the drop landings, ground reaction forces, EMG and kinematics were recorded. The EMG and the ground reaction forces were synchronised by means of a TTL signal which was fed onto both data acquisition boards. Simultaneously four parallel switched light emitting diodes lighted up. These served to synchronize the cameras with each other and with the remaining systems.

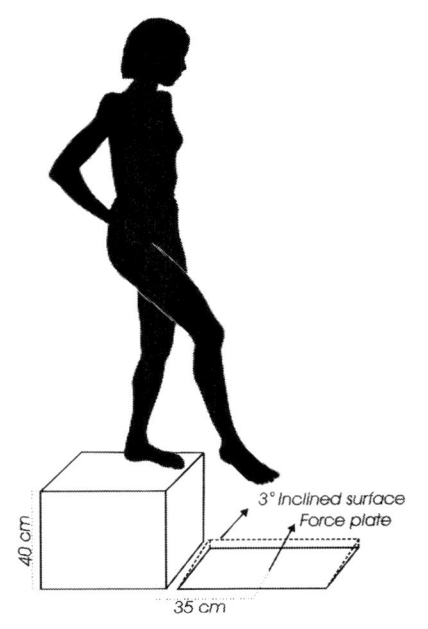

Figure 4.1.
Schematic representation of the experimental set up: The subjects had to perform one legged drop landings onto three different surfaces: A level one and two surfaces inclined 3 degrees either laterally or medially. The subjects were instructed to land on their left foot and stabilise their body as soon as possible. The drop was initiated by forwarding the right foot and pushing off from the box with the left one having the leg almost completely extended. The hands were held on the hips.

Ground reaction forces

The ground reaction forces were recorded at 1000 Hz by means of a forceplate (Kistler, type: 9881B21, Winterthur, Switzerland) embedded into the floor. The landing surfaces were fixed (securely screwed) onto the plate. The centre of the plate was 35 cm in front of the edge of the starting box (Figure 4.1). This distance proved to be the mean distance from the box at which the subjects landed centred onto the plate. The instant of TD was determined from the ground reaction force data when the vertical force exceeded 20 N. The three components of the ground reaction force data were analysed separately.

Electromyography

Bipolar, preamplified (analogue RC-filter 10–500 Hz bandwidth) surface electrodes (Biovision, Wehrheim, Germany) with an interelectrode distance of 2 cm were used for EMG collection. The signals from 6 muscles of the lower leg: peroneus longus, peroneus brevis, soleus, lateral gastrocnemius, medial gastrocnemius, and tibialis anterior were sampled at 1000 Hz.

Despite no artefacts were detected by passive leg shaking or by slight hopping after preparation, in several cases artefacts appeared synchronously with TD during both inclined conditions. These could be removed without substantial alteration of the remaining signal by high pass filtering the signals at 30 Hz cut off frequency. This was done for all EMG signals. Afterwards, the curves were smoothed by means of a 30 points back and forth moving root mean square algorithm in order to allow a point-by-point comparison of the EMG (see data analysis at the end of the methods section). No time shift was introduced neither by the filtering nor by the smoothing.

Kinematics

Foot motion was captured by 4 cameras: Two operating at 120 Hz (60/120 Hz NTSC, Peak Performance Technologies, Inc. Centennial, CO–USA) and two operating at 250 Hz (one Redlake 250C and one KODAK Motion Corder Analyzer SR-500c, Roper Scientific MASD, SanDiego, CA-USA). The video data were digitised using the MOTUS 6 software (Peak Performance Technologies, Inc. Centennial, CO-USA). After obtaining the 3D coordinates from each camera pair, the data were interpolated using quintic splines to achieve a common frequency (1000 Hz).

The lower leg and the foot were modelled by means of a multi-body system, comprising 4 rigid bodies (Arampatzis et al., 2002 and 2003) (Figure 4.2). The calculations were done using the simulation software "alaska" (advanced lagrangian solver in kinetic analysis, version 3.0,

Chemnitz, Germany). The model considers the motion between rearfoot and shank (from now on referred to as ankle joint), the medial column of the forefoot to the rearfoot (from now on referred to as medial foot joint), and the lateral column of the forefoot to the rearfoot (from now on referred to as lateral foot joint). The motion at the ankle joint includes both, the motion at the tibiotalar and the subtalar joints. The motion calculated for the medial foot joint corresponds to the sum of the motion of all structures included in the medial forefoot. In the same manner, the motion of the lateral foot joint corresponds to the motion of all structures included in the lateral forefoot. Due to these simplifications the model does not describe the true motion of the foot bones. However, the model tried to account for the functional anatomy of the foot and allows the examination of the kinematics in a more functional way than simpler models.

Model definition: For each joint, two joint coordinate systems attached to each of the connected segments were defined. The joint coordinate systems were defined in a neutral position (Figure 4.2): Subject seated, knee angle at 90°, tibia to floor 90° (in the sagittal and in the frontal plane), longitudinal axis of the foot contained in the sagittal plane. Seventeen reflective skin mounted markers were attached to the left shank and foot of the subjects (Table 4.1, Figure 4.2). Eight markers were fixed on predefined anatomical landmarks to allow the definition of the joint coordinate systems. Nine more markers were placed on not strictly defined anatomical positions but rather on locations where lesser skin movements were expected. Five markers (1, 2, 4, 7 and 8) were only needed for the model definition and were detached for the landings. Inversely to the original model from Arampatzis et al. (2002 and 2003), in the present one, marker 3 (most medial point of the tuberositas naviculare) was kept for dynamic tracking. A marker on the instep above the Os naviculare utilised in the original model was not used. This was done because marker 3 showed to be more stable during movement than the marker on the instep above the Os naviculare.

The kinematics of the ankle, the medial and the lateral foot joints, were defined by the orientation of the most distal joint coordinate system with respect to the more proximal one. Eversion-inversion, dorsi-plantar flexion and adduction-abduction were defined utilising the Bryant angles describing the rotations about the corresponding axis for each motion.

A more detailed description of the model can be found in Arampatzis et al. 2002 and 2003.

Table 4.1. *Markers used to define and steer the foot and shank model.*

Bony landmarks	Other markers
1. Caput metatarsale I (most medial point)	9. Caput metatarsale I (medial superior)
2. Caput metatarsale V (most lateral point)	10. Caput metatarsale V (lateral superior)
3. Tuberositas naviculare (most medial point)	11. Caput metatarsale II-III (between 2nd & 3rd metatarsal heads)
4. Os Cuboideum (diagonal superior to the basis of the 5th metatarsal)	12. Metatarsus I (more proximal)
5. Malleolus medialis (most medial point)	13. Metatarsus V (more proximal)
6. Malleolus lateralis (most lateral point)	14. Calcaneus medial (more anterior)
7. Condilus medialis tibiae (most medial point)	15. Calcaneus medial (more posterior)
8. Caput fibula (most lateral point)	16. Calcaneus lateral
	17. Fascies tibiae

The bony landmarks are used to define the model, whereas the other markers are only needed to track the motion. See also figure 4.2.

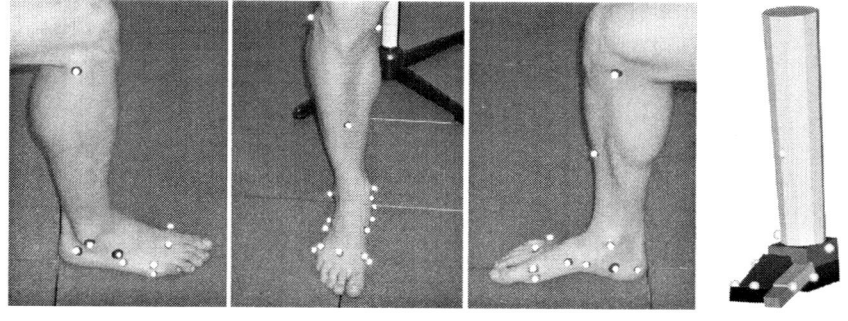

Figure 4.2. *Lateral, frontal and medial view of the foot and shank with all markers fixed, as it is placed for the reference measurement. At the right side a view of the model. For this study only four rigid bodies were considered: Shank, rearfoot, medial forefoot and lateral forefoot.*

For most subjects one of the markers defining the medial column of the forefoot could not be tracked accurately during the first phase of the whole landing. There were not enough data to perform statistics regarding the motion of the medial foot joint during this phase. Therefore, for this joint results are presented only from 60 ms after TD on.

Data analysis

After visual inspection of all curves, three trials per condition from each subject were averaged. This way we obtained 24 mean curves, for each condition and parameter: mediolateral, antero-posterior, and vertical GRF, EMG from each of the six muscles, and eversion-inversion, dorsi-plantarflexion and adduction-abduction motion for each of the three considered joints. The kinematics were available only for 21 subjects. An analysis of variance for repeated measures was performed millisecond by millisecond for each of the parameters to test the influence of the landing surface. The level of significance was set to $p<0.05$. Then a Bonferroni adjusted pairwise comparison between the different surface conditions was done millisecond by millisecond for each parameter. The level of significance was set to $p<0.05$.

In order to describe the magnitude of the differences between conditions the root mean square differences between the means of each subject were calculated for every millisecond. For considering a difference as meaningful it had to be above certain threshold: In the case of the ground reaction forces and the EMG signals the root mean square difference had to be above 10% of the maximal value of the corresponding mean curve obtained for the level condition. This threshold was arbitrarily chosen as in clinical diagnostic, differences below 10% are often considered as normal deviations. For the kinematics an absolute threshold of 2 degrees was taken. This was done based on the typical differences found between stable and unstable ankles in joint position sense tests (Konradsen, 2002).

4.3 Results

Ground reaction forces

Figure 4.3 shows the mean curves of the ground reaction forces as well as the significant differences being greater than 10% of the corresponding maximum force on the level surface. The shape of the curves was in general quite similar for all three conditions. Most of the significant differences ($p<0.05$) were greater than the threshold. The absolute thresholds for relevant differences were 4.1 N/Kg, 0.3 N/Kg and 0.6 N/Kg for the vertical, the mediolateral and the antero-posterior forces respectively.

For the medio-lateral forces most of the differences appeared during the first 0–50 ms. Differences between the inclined surfaces were more frequent than between the level and the inclined ones. Trials onto the laterally inclined surface had higher lateral forces, followed by the level and finally the medially inclined one. In the same manner trials onto the medially inclined surface had higher medially directed forces. For the antero-posterior forces the differences between the level and the inclined surfaces were scarce, showing lower posterior forces onto the level surface immediately after TD. In contrast no differences between the inclined conditions were detected prior to 43 ms after TD. From then on a considerable amount of differences was observed between both

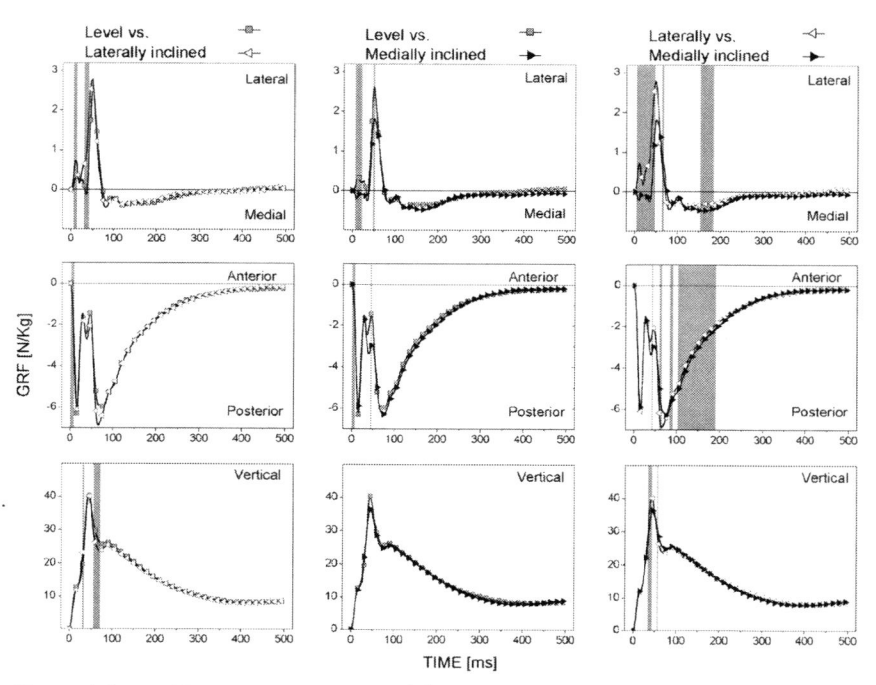

Figure 4.3.   *Mean curves (n=24) of the ground reaction forces during landings onto three different surfaces: Level, 3° lateral inclination, 3° medial inclination. The shaded areas indicate significant differences (p<0.05) being greater than 10% of the maximal value at the level condition.*

inclined conditions up to almost 200 ms post TD. Differences between the lateral and the other two surface conditions in the vertical GRF appeared within the first 75 ms after TD. In general the ground reaction forces showed somewhat smoother patterns for the landings onto the medially inclined surface. This was especially true for the mediolateral forces during the first 50 ms, but also for the vertical impact force which was 10% lower onto the medially inclined surface than onto the laterally inclined one.

Electromyography

The mean curves representing the EMG patterns for the different conditions can be seen in figures 4.4 and 4.5. Almost all of the significant dif-

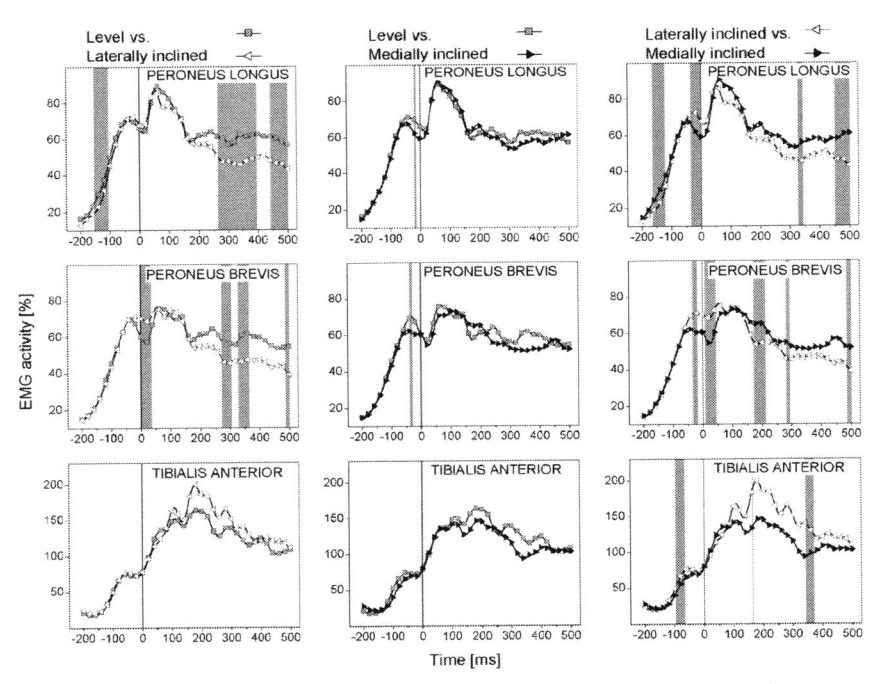

Figure 4.4. Mean curves (n=24) of the EMG envelopes during landings onto three different surfaces: Level, 3° lateral inclination, 3° medial inclination. The shaded areas indicate significant differences (p<0.05) being greater than 10% of the maximal value at the level condition.

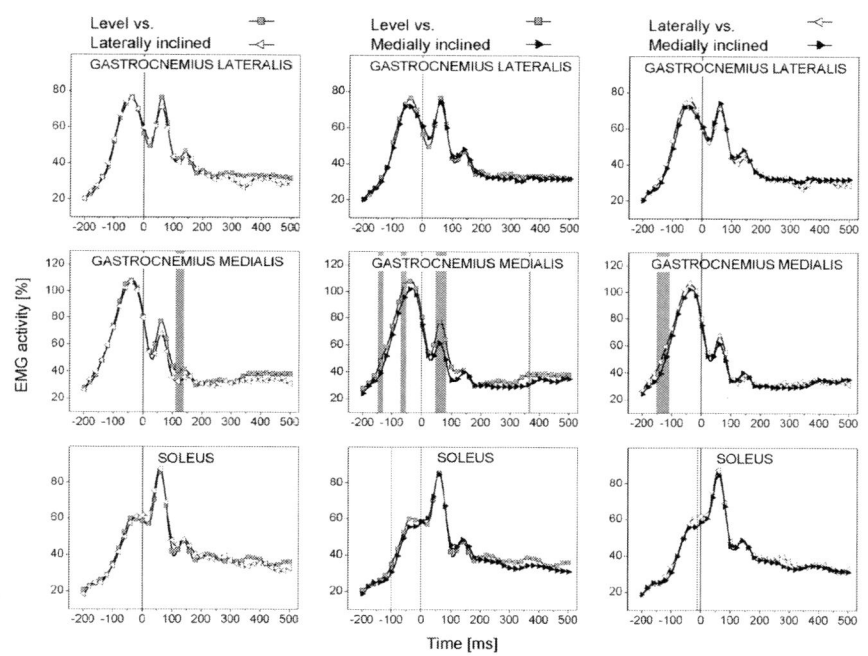

Foot and ankle stabilisation during drop landing 87

Figure 4.5. Mean curves (n=24) of the EMG envelopes during landings onto three different surfaces: Level, 3° lateral inclination, 3° medial inclination. The shaded areas indicate significant differences ($p<0.05$) being greater than 10% of the maximal value at the level condition.

ferences ($p<0.05$) were greater than the 10% threshold. The peroneal muscles behaved significantly different ($p<0.05$) in all three conditions even prior to TD (Figure 4.4). The differences appearing in close proximity, prior or after TD indicated highest peroneal activities onto the laterally inclined surface followed by the level surface and finally the medially inclined one. These differences were often reversed later in time. For the tibialis anterior the significant differences indicated lower activity levels onto the medially inclined surface than onto the laterally inclined one; however no significant differences appeared near TD.

The behaviour of the triceps surae muscles can be observed in figure 4.5. The lateral gastrocnemius was not significantly ($p>0.05$) affected by the different surface conditions. There were no significant differences prior to TD for any of the triceps surae muscles between the level and the lateral condition. For the soleus the only significant differences between conditions were very discrete in time and appeared prior to TD. In contrast to the other two heads of the triceps surae, the medial gastrocnemius was significantly ($p<0.05$) influenced by the different surface conditions, showing lower values ($p<0.05$) prior to TD onto the medially inclined surface and after TD higher values ($p<0.05$) onto the level surface.

Kinematics

In figures 4.6, 4.7 and 4.8 the mean curves of the motion around each axis as well as the significant differences ($p<0.05$) between landing conditions being greater than 2°, are presented for all 3 studied joints. The results concerning the medial foot joint were only available from 60 ms after TD on (see methods section). Prior to TD only the lateral foot joint showed significant differences ($p<0.05$), namely for the eversion-inversion motion (Figure 4.6). At both forefoot joints the eversion-inversion motion pattern reflected an adaptation to the ground. The patterns were significantly different ($p<0.05$) for all surfaces during almost the whole analysed time window. These joints were most everted during landings onto the medially inclined surface, followed by the level surface and finally the laterally inclined one. The different surfaces caused a mean shift in the ordinates, which exceeded by about one degree the differences in surface inclination: For the lateral foot joint the shifts were 4.0° between the level and the laterally inclined surface, 4.1° between level and medially inclined, and 8.1° between both inclined surfaces; for the medial foot joint the corresponding values were 3.6°, 3.4° and 7.1°. For the eversion-inversion motion the ankle joint displayed significant differences only around 50 ms after TD, where the medially inclined surface led to higher eversion values.

When comparing the dorsiflexion-plantarflexion motion among the different conditions (Figure 4.7) the ankle showed higher dorsiflexion values onto the level surface than onto the laterally inclined one, approximately for the 2nd 75 ms. The medial foot joint behaved very similar onto the level and the laterally inclined surfaces during the first 250 ms. Later on, the dorsiflexion values were higher ($p<0.05$) onto the laterally inclined surface. Onto the medially inclined surface this joint showed significantly lower dorsiflexion values throughout the whole available data. In contrast, the dorsiflexion-plantarflexion behaviour of the lateral foot joint seemed not to be affected by the different surface conditions.

The plots of the adduction-abduction motion (Figure 4.8) show no significant differences above two degrees among the tested surface conditions, neither for the ankle nor for the medial foot joint. The lateral foot joint displayed significantly higher abduction values (p<0.05) around 25 ms post TD onto the laterally inclined surface compared to the other surfaces.

In general, for the kinematics the standard deviations were highest near TD, especially for the adduction-abduction motion, indicating interindividual differences in initial landing position. Later on the standard deviations were somewhat lower and quite stable.

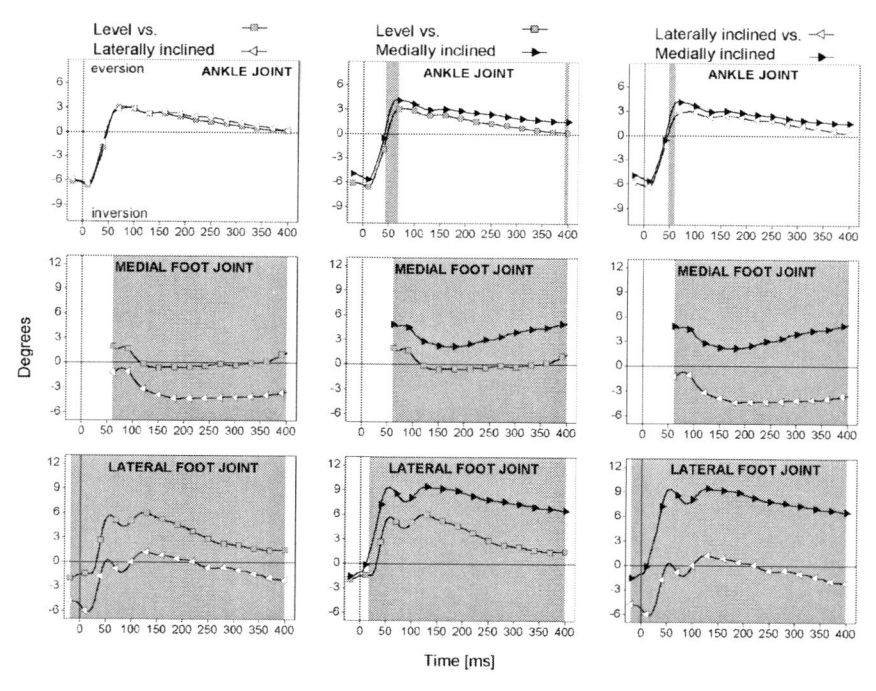

Figure 4.6. *Mean curves (n=21) representing the eversion inversion motion of the different joints considered in the model during landings onto three different surfaces: Level, 3° lateral inclination, 3° medial inclination. The shaded areas indicate significant differences (p<0.05) being greater than 2°.*

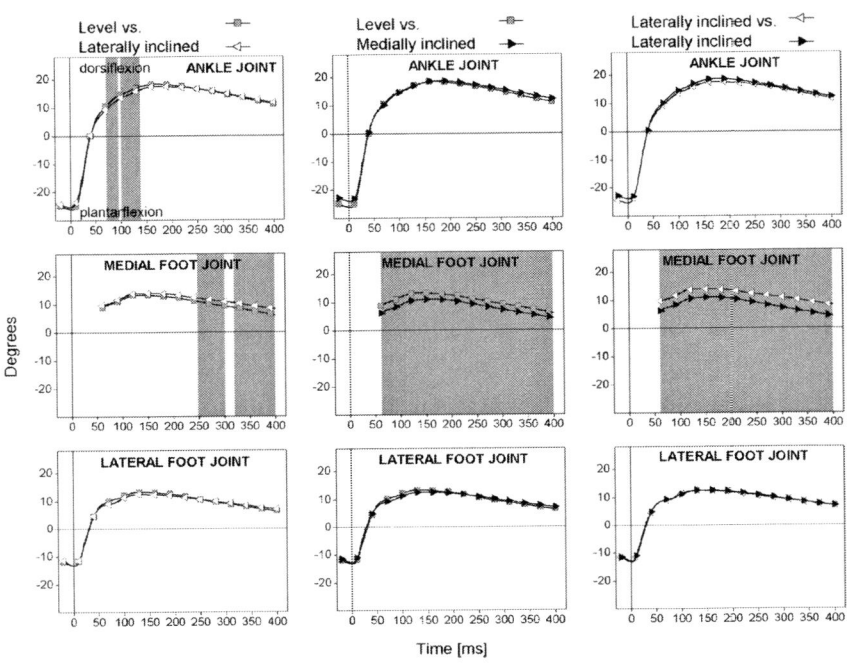

Figure 4.7. Mean curves (n=21) representing the dorsiflexion-plantarflexion motion of the different joints considered in the model during landings onto three different surfaces: Level, 3° lateral inclination, 3° medial inclination. The shaded areas indicate significant differences ($p<0.05$) being greater than 2°.

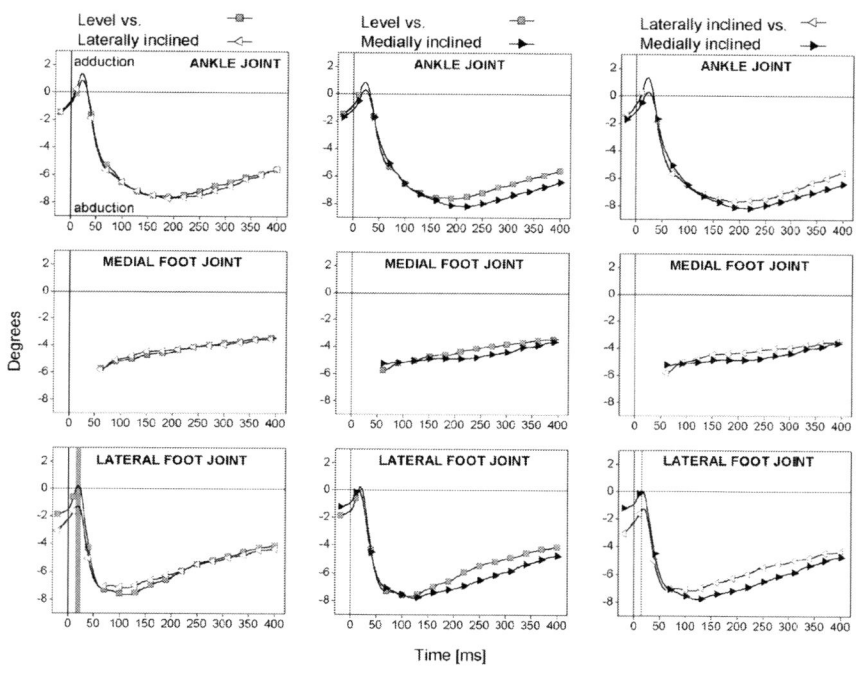

Figure 4.8. Mean curves (n=21) representing the adduction-abduction motion of the different joints considered in the model during landings onto three different surfaces: Level, 3° lateral inclination, 3° medial inclination. The shaded areas indicate significant differences (p<0.05) being greater than 2°.

4.4 Discussion

The three experimental conditions differed by 3 and 6 degrees in frontal plane surface inclination. Whereas the forefoot joints adapt to the surface inclination as seen by a corresponding shift in the eversion-inversion pattern, the ankle joint demonstrates very low shifts and only a few significant differences in ankle eversion-inversion patterns between the medially inclined condition and the other two surfaces (Figure 4.6). All kinematic, EMG and GRF patterns were similar for the three conditions. Nevertheless several significant, surface specific differences were observed prior and after TD. Next the results of this study will be discussed regarding the origin and functionality of the observed patterns in adapting to the different surface conditions.

The EMG plots (Figures 4.4 and 4.5) reflect the result of the central motor commands and the modulations due to reflex mechanisms triggered by the interaction between subject and landing surface. During landing, the main sources of feedback discerning between surfaces are the GRF and the kinematics imposed after TD. The interplay of these commands with the environmental and anatomical configurations will produce the observed kinematics which in turn will influence the GRF and possibly again the following EMG.

The surface specific differences observed prior to TD indicate feedforward adjustments to the landing condition. So the kinematic data reveal that the foot position is adjusted according to surface inclination, as shown by the higher inversion of the lateral forefoot at TD when landing onto the laterally inclined surface (Figure 4.6). Foot position at TD can be crucial for the subsequent stabilisation, as a different joint configuration changes the geometry of the foot and of the subsequent collision with the ground (Wright et al., 2000). Furthermore the potential of passive (bony and ligamentous) and active (muscles) structures to counteract the imminent destabilising forces can be changed by altering their orientation and hence their lever arms to the joint axes or their tension. This means that the destabilising moments occurring at TD as well as the potential of the biological system to cope with them may be influenced prior to TD. A correct prediction of the disturbance to come would therefore allow a better adjustment of the involved structures before the foot touches the ground.

The earliest differences observed in the EMG (more than 100 ms prior to TD, Figures 4.4 and 4.5), when most of the muscles show a relatively low activation, might be related to foot positioning. So, the higher lateral forefoot (probably also medial forefoot) inversion at TD seen for the laterally inclined surface condition (Figure 4.6), could be related to the lower activity at the peroneus longus 100 to 150 ms prior to TD at this condition. Pre-activation levels immediately prior to TD (last 100 or 50 ms), when most muscles around the joint show a considerable activation level, have been typically associated to muscle stiffness regulation (Arampatzis et al., 2001a, b). During landings the aim is to bring the carried energy to zero. During the first 40 to 60 ms the GRF are especially high. Therefore, an appropriate tuning of muscle stiffness at TD is important. Our data show both peroneal muscles being more active just prior to TD when landing onto the laterally inclined surface compared to the medially inclined one (Figure 4.4). This suggests the need of tuning these muscles stiffer for this condition.

Evidence for central feedforward adjustments to landing onto different surfaces and from different heights has been previously reported (McKinley and Pedotti, 1992; Arampatzis et al., 2003). McKinley and Pedotti (1992) observed a shift in the EMG onset times towards TD when instead of a rigid surface, a foam surface was expected. Furthermore, they found skilled subjects to have a higher plantarflexion angle at TD when landing onto the rigid surface as compared to foam. Arampatzis et al. (2003) found increased EMG prior and after TD with increasing falling height when landing onto gymnastic mats. In contrast Grüneberg et al. (2003) reported no differences in pre-activity on the peroneus longus or the soleus, albeit considerably higher differences in frontal plane inclination (0° vs. 25° inverting platform) as compared to the present study. This apparent discrepancy can rely onto how pre-activation was quantified. The authors quantified pre-activity as a mean value during a 50 ms window prior to TD, whereas in the present study we observed each millisecond for 200 ms prior to TD. Furthermore in the present study the same muscles (peroneus longus and soleus) did not show significant differences in the 50 ms prior to TD either, when comparing level with laterally inclined surface trials.

The higher EMG activity of the peroneus brevis onto the laterally inclined surface observed early after TD (within the first 40 ms) can not arise from any reflex elicited at the instant of collision since there is not enough time available. On one hand lowered H-reflexes at TD have been described for the soleus during landings (Dyhre-Poulsen et al., 1991) indicating that reflexes would have no substantial effect at this time. On the other hand, except for the tibialis anterior, the shortest reported latencies of lower leg muscles during landings are slightly above 40 ms (Grüneberg et al., 2003; Duncan and McDonagh, 2000). Furthermore Grüneberg et al. (2003) found these early responses to be very unspecific. Specific long latency responses took about 90 ms to appear; almost 50 ms after the plate had reached its final position. Therefore, the post-TD differences observed within the first 50 ms in EMG for the peroneus brevis (Figure 4.4), as well as those in the kinematics (Figure 4.6 and 4.8) or the GRF (Figure 4.3) result from the differing initial conditions, i.e. different surface inclination and different surface specific feedforward adjustments (foot position at TD and muscle stiffness).

The existing literature has mainly focused on the neural aspect of active joint stabilisation and only secondary attention has been paid to the passive stabilising mechanisms. These latter however, seem to play the main role during the early phase of the collision, when the acting forces are highest. During this phase the neural system has no time to produce any reactive command. These should have already been made in a feedforward manner prior to TD in order to create adequate conditions for the passive mechanisms to work properly. So it seems as if to cope with landings onto the laterally inclined condition a higher forefoot inversion at TD and a higher activation level of the peroneal muscles is advantageous. For the medially inclined surface, during the first 40 ms after TD the mediolateral forces remained fairly close to zero and also the vertical force maximum was lower as compared to the laterally inclined surface (Figure 4.3). At the same time the eversion-inversion amplitude of the lateral forefoot was considerably higher for this condition (Figure 4.6). These data suggest that higher eversion amplitudes provide certain damping. The fact that the peroneus brevis was significantly less active during this period for this condition, further suggests that the additional damping is achieved in a passive manner.

We would suggest that the positioning of the lateral forefoot (possibly also the medial one) prior to TD produces a joint configuration such that the lever arms and the passive constraints are more propitious for the subsequent stabilisation onto a given surface. For the landing tasks studied here, the aim of the adjustments anticipating the consequences of the surface condition might be to try to take the best advantage of the physiological and anatomical self-stabilizing properties of the musculoskeletal system. So when landing onto the medially inclined surface, the lateral forefoot is placed closer to the neutral eversion-inversion position at TD (Figure 4.6). This probably leads to a lower everting moment of the GRF, and places the foot in a position where the passive constraints to eversion will act sooner. This would be advantageous to cope with the landing task and relief the neuromuscular system, since the contribution of passive mechanisms to joint stabilisation would be enhanced.

The presented results support the idea that the biological system tries to enhance its self-stabilizing capability prior to TD. Self-stabilising mechanisms are not new in the literature. Katz (1939) showed that activated muscles respond to rapid stretches with an immediate increase in force generation due to their force-velocity characteristic, reaching values up to 200% of their maximal isometric force. This provides a zero delay stabilising mechanism, which Loeb (1995) termed as preflex. The idea of stabilising preflexes has been extended to passive dynamics, i.e. early stabilisation reactions that arise solely from the passive interaction between the anatomical structures and the external forces, for example by varying lever arms (Moritz and Farley, 2004; Wagner and Blickhan, 2003).

Motor commands arising from the feedback after TD have the possibility to participate in the stabilisation process later on. First specific reflex stabilising responses can be expected from 90 ms post TD on (Grüneberg et al., 2003). At this time also voluntary central commands triggered by post TD information may reach the leg and also modulate the reflex responses (Grüneberg et al., 2003). In the present study both peroneal muscles, as well as the tibialis anterior and the gastrocnemius medialis show surface specific activation patterns later than 100 ms. At this time the ground reaction forces have already reached their maximum and tend towards zero (or towards bodyweight in the case of the vertical forces). Further differences in EMG appeared even later than 200 ms post TD, when all joints have reached their maximum and the rotations are relatively slow. Therefore it is suggested that these adjustments are rather related to the maintenance of balance, than to counteract the destabilising forces caused by the collision with the ground.

Most recent authors (Nielsen, 2004; Santello, 2005) support the idea that motor commands are steered according to the expected interactions with the environment. This is in accordance with the adjustments observed in EMG and in the kinematics prior to TD at the present study. Our proprioceptive system is responsible for the continuous survey of the agreement between the expected and the actual consequences of this interaction. Discrepancies i.e. presence or absence of expected feedback, should be detected and lead to the pertinent adjustments (Nielsen, 2004). However, because of the inherent latencies associated to feedback mechanisms, the feedback originated adjustments are in general not effective for preventing acute injuries or perturbations (Isakov et al., 1986; Konradsen et al., 1997). Therefore several authors suggest that proprioception is more related to learning than to the acute control of sudden perturbations (Gauffin et al., 1988; Flanagan et al., 2003). This way, appropriate motor commands can be produced for subsequent interactions (Patton et al., 2000; Marigold and Patla, 2002).

Concluding: Our results show that feedforward strategies were present. However, repeated motor tasks are never identical and feedforward strategies alone are probably insufficient to provide an adequate adaptation to this variability. The results further indicate that when landing onto different surfaces, feedforward strategies try to set up the most favourable conditions for the self-stabilising mechanisms of the musculoskeletal system to work properly. This can bridge the interval (first 40-90 ms) where feedback mechanisms can not produce a specific response, and also reduce the later need to rely on feedback information for a successful task completion. Furthermore it seems as if the increased eversion-inversion amplitude of the lateral forefoot caused by the 3° medial surface inclination can be related to a damping mechanism, relieving the neuromuscular system as indicated by the lower EMG activity together with the slightly smoother ground reaction forces. At last, the background presented here could explain the effectiveness of rehabilitation programmes, even in presence of proprioceptive deficits, since more adequate feedforward adjustments could be learned, leading to an enhanced self-stabilisation and hence reducing the need of relying on possibly impaired or reduced feedback information.

4.5 References

Arampatzis, A.; Brüggemann, G.-P.; Morey Klapsing, G. (2001a). Leg stiffness and mechanical energetic processes during jumping on a sprung surface. Medicine and Science in Sports and Exercise 33, 923–931

Arampatzis, A.; Brüggemann, G.-P.; Morey Klapsing, G.M. (2002). A three-dimensional shank-foot model to determine the foot motion during landings. Medicine and Science in Sports and Exercise 34, 130–138

Arampatzis, A.; Morey Klapsing, G.M.; Brüggemann, G.-P. (2003). The effect of falling height on muscle activity and foot motion during landings. Journal of Electromyography and Kinesiology 13, 533–544

Arampatzis, A.; Schade, F.; Walsh, M.; Brüggemann, G.-P. (2001b). Influence of leg stiffness and its effect on myodynamic jumping performance. Journal of Electromyography and Kinesiology 11, 355–364

Caulfield, B.M.; Garrett, M. (2002). Functional instability of the ankle: Differences in patterns of ankle and knee movement prior to and post landing in a single leg jump. International Journal of Sports Medicine 23, 64–68

Caulfield, B.M.; Garrett, M. (2004). Changes in ground reaction force during jump landing in subjects with functional instability of the ankle joint. Clinical Biomechanics 19, 617–621

Caster, B.L.; Bates, B.T. (1995). The assessment of mechanical and neuromuscular response strategies during landing. Medicine and Science in Sports and Exercise 27: 736–744

Dufek, J.S.; Bates, B.T. (1990). The evaluation and prediction of impact forces during landings. Medicine and Science in Sports and Exercise 22, 370–377

Duncan, A.; McDonagh, M.J. (2000). Stretch reflex distinguished from pre-programmed muscle activations following landing impacts in man. Journal of Physiology 526, 457–568

Dyhre-Poulsen, P. Mosfeldt Laursen, A. (1984). Programmed electromyographic activity and negative incremental muscle stiffness in monkeys jumping downward. Journal of Physiology 350, 121–136

Dyhre-Poulsen, P.; Simonsen, E.B.; Voigt, M. (1991). Dynamic control of muscle stiffness and H reflex modulation during hopping and jumping in man. Journal of Physiology 437, 287–304

Flanagan, J.R.; Vetter, P.; Johansson, R.S.; Wolpert, D.M. (2003). Prediction precedes control in motor learning. Current Biology 13. 146–150

Gauffin, H.; Tropp, H.; Odenrick, P. (1988). Effect of ankle disk training on postural control in patients with functional instability of the ankle joint. Journal of Sports Medicine 9, 141–144

Gross, T.S.; Nelson, R.C. (1988). The shock attenuation role of the ankle during landing from a vertical jump. Medicine and Science in Sports and Exercise 20, 506–514

Grüneberg, C.; Nieuwenhuijzen, P.H.; Duysens, J. (2003). Reflex responses in the lower leg following landing impact on an inverting and non-inverting platform. Journal of Physiology 550, 985–993

Isakov, E.; Mizrahi, J.; Solzi, P.; Susak, Z.; Lotem, M. (1986). Response of the peroneal muscles to sudden inversion of the ankle during standing. International Journal of Sports Biomechanics 2, 100–109

Katz, B. (1939). The relation between force and speed in muscular contraction. Journal of Physiology 96, 45–64

Konradsen, L. (2002). Factors contributing to chronic ankle instability: Kinesthesia and joint position sense. Journal of Athletic Training 37, 381–385

Konradsen, L.; Voigt, M.; Hojsgaard, C. (1997). Ankle inversion injuries. The role of the dynamic defense mechanism. American Journal of Sports Medicine 25, 54–58

Liebermann, D.G.; Hoffman, J.R. (2005). Timing of preparatory landing responses as a function of availability of optic flow information. Journal of Electromyography and Kinesiology 15, 120–130

Loeb, G.E. (1995). Control implications of musculoskeletal mechanics. Book of abstracts of the Annual International Conference of the IEEE-EMBS 17, 1393–1394

Marigold, D.S.; Patla, A.E. (2002). Strategies for dynamic stability during locomotion on a slippery surface: effects of prior experience and knowledge. Journal of Neurophysiology 88: 339–353

McKinley, P.; Pedotti, A. (1992). Motor strategies in landing from a jump: the role of skill in task execution. Experimental Brain Research 90, 427–440

Moritz, C.T.; Farley, C.T. (2004). Passive dynamics change leg mechanics for an unexpected surface during human hopping. Journal of Applied Physiology 97, 1313–1322

Nielsen, J.B. (2004). Sensorimotor integration at spinal level as a basis for muscle coordination during voluntary movement in humans. Journal of Applied Physiology 96, 1961–1967

Patton, J.L.; Lee, W.A.; Pai, Y.C. (2000). Relative stability improves with experience in a dynamic standing task. Experimental Brain Research 135, 117–126

Pelland, L.; McKinley, P. (2004). A pattern recognition technique to characterize the differential modulation of co-activating muscles at the performer/environment interface. Journal of Electromyography and Kinesiology 14, 539–554

Santello, M. (2005). Review of motor control mechanisms underlying impact absorption from falls. Gait Posture 21, 85–94

Santello, M.; McDonagh, M.J. (1998). The control of timing and amplitude of EMG activity in landing movements in humans. Experimental Physiology 83, 857–874

Self, B.P.; Paine, D. (2001). Ankle biomechanics during four landing techniques. Medicine and Science in Sports and Exercise 33, 1338–1344

Stacoff, A.; Kaelin, X.; Stuessi, E.; Segesser, B. (1990). Die Torsionsbewegung des Fußes beim Landen nach einem Sprung. Zeitschrift für Orthopädie und Ihre Grenzgebiete 128, 213–217

Stacoff, A.; Reinschmidt, C.; Nigg, B.M.; van den Bogert, A.J.; Lundberg, A.; Denoth, J.; Stüssi, E. (2000). Effects of foot orthoses on skeletal motion during running. Clinical Biomechanics 15, 54–64

Thompson, H.W.; McKinley, P.A. (1995). Landing from a jump: the role of vision when landing from known and unknown heights. Neuro Report 6, 581–584

Wagner, H.; Blickhan, R. (2003). Stabilizing function of antagonistic neuromusculoskeletal systems: an analytical investigation. Biological Cybernetics 89, 71–79

Wright, I.C.; Neptune, R.R.; van den Bogert, A.J.; Nigg, B.M. (2000). The influence of foot positioning on ankle sprains. Journal of Biomechanics 33, 513–519

Summary and Conclusions

Probably one of the main contributions of this thesis has been the use of a three-dimensional kinematic model accounting not only for ankle motion but also for the motion of the lateral and medial columns of the forefoot with regard to the rearfoot (Arampatzis et al., 2002), in a joint stability context. The obtained values may serve as reference for the planning of further studies and provide a base for building up new hypotheses. However this thesis did not aim to merely describe the kinematics but rather to provide more knowledge regarding the stabilisation of the foot and the ankle. Therefore another important contribution is surely the simultaneous study of the kinematics, the EMG and the ground reaction forces, which allows a better understanding of the whole stabilisation process.

The presented results have shown that forefoot motion is fundamental in foot and ankle stabilisation. The flexibility of the forefoot, especially in the frontal plane, permits a fast and appropriate adaptation to the ground. Furthermore the high mobility of the forefoot, allows the ankle to rotate slower and to a lesser extent. Possibly this reduction in required ankle motion can contribute considerably to injury prevention, since the forces acting at the ankle are high and a misalignment with regard to the ground reaction forces could rapidly lead to moments overwhelming the stabilising potential of the involved structures. In addition, the rapid adaptation of the forefoot to the ground can potentially provide more precise and earlier feedback regarding the ground characteristics than the structures surrounding the ankle joint. This way the corresponding adjustments in an immediate feedback could happen earlier, and the consequences of future interactions could be predicted more accurately.

The results from the presented studies support the notion that joint stabilisation does not rely primarily on proprioception. Prolonged peroneal latencies might in fact be due to deafferentiation consequent to the recurrent sprains. However prolonged latencies do not seem to be responsible for a functional instability. On one hand the differences in latency times between healthy and unstable ankles are relatively low and not consistently observed. Those studies identifying prolonged latencies in functionally unstable joints, report differences close to 15 ms (Konradsen and Ravn, 1990; Löfvenberg et al., 1995). Fifteen ms is a short time to have a high functional impact on joint stabilisation. Furthermore the presented results strongly suggest that the temporal characteristics of the EMG response play a less important role than those related to EMG amplitude. Finally, healthy or not, the latencies are in general too long to provide reactive protection against strong sudden perturbations. During the inverting tilt plate tests the EMG activity during the first 50 ms is almost negligible, but both forefoot joints are almost maximally inverted. In addition the highest mediolateral ground reaction forces occur as soon as 25 ms after plate release. So during these first milliseconds, the stabilisation has to rely onto passive mechanisms. At the sudden everting tilts, the EMG activity shows the same temporal pattern as inverting tilts, but lower amplitudes. At the same time the kinematics are in general lower in amplitude and velocity. These findings together with the higher passive constraints to eversion than to inversion (Siegler et al., 1994) underpin the importance of passive constraints during the early phase of recovery from a sudden disturbance.

Awareness has shown to improve stabilisation even when no differences in activation prior to plate release were identified. On the other hand it has been shown that the early reactive response to a joint perturbation is unspecific in nature (similar EMG patterns despite of opposite disturbance directions). Accordingly Grüneberg et al. (2003) found specific responses to appear relatively late in time (~90 ms). Finally specific adaptive responses to an expected perturbation are given in a feedforward manner (specific changes in joint positioning and activation according to landing surface). All these findings together suggest that experience may play a crucial role in joint stabilisation. The more experience we have the better we can anticipate the effects of the next interaction with the environment. Consequently the anticipative adjustments would be more adequate. Nevertheless it has also been shown that it is possible to stabilise the foot and ankle joints despite of not being aware of the instant of tilt. The consequences are higher ground reaction forces and higher needed muscular activation levels. As discussed somewhat earlier, these higher activation levels would probably be too late in absence of other stabilising mechanisms. Moritz and Farley (2004) found adaptive stabilising responses to surprising changes in surface stiffness prior to identifiable changes in the EMG. These changes were due to the passive dynamics inherent to the anatomy and physiology of our musculoskeletal system, which seems to include self-stabilising mechanisms in its design (Wagner and Blickhan, 2003). When observing all the presented results together, it can be suggested with reasonable evidence, that experience and awareness can improve the usage of the self-stabilising mechanisms. It is suggested that the observed proactive adjustments aim to produce the best suited conditions (segmental orientation and muscle tension) to cope with the perturbation to come. The proved effectiveness of proprioceptive training in the rehabilitation of functionally unstable joints (Verhagen et al., 2000) can also be explained by the presented theoretical frame, without the need of assuming that stabilisation strongly relies on proprioception. The repeated experience would provide the information necessary for a better and even earlier prediction of the consequences of the next interaction. It could further help to generate more suited default strategies for the case of being surprised.

Although not experimentally proven, there is a general consensus on that severe ankle sprains usually happen because the foot is brought into a position where even fully activated muscles cannot resist the injuring moment. The only way for avoiding such extreme positions is to prevent them in advance. Accordingly Eils and Rosenbaum (2003) suggested, that the main function of braces is not the restriction of motion in acute situations, but holding the foot in a position where it is unlikely to elicit such extreme situations. This way sprains are mainly prevented rather than counteracted.

BIBLIOGRAPHY

Arampatzis, A.; Brüggemann, G.-P.; Morey Klapsing, G. (2001a). Leg stiffness and mechanical energetic processes during jumping on a sprung surface. Medicine and Science in Sports and Exercise 33, 923–931

Arampatzis, A.; Brüggemann, G.-P.; Morey Klapsing, G.M. (2002). A three-dimensional shank-foot model to determine the foot motion during landings. Medicine and Science in Sports and Exercise 34, 130–138

Arampatzis, A.; Morey Klapsing, G.M.; Brüggemann, G.-P. (2003). The effect of falling height on muscle activity and foot motion during landings. Journal of Electromyography and Kinesiology 13, 533–544

Arampatzis, A.; Schade, F.; Walsh, M.; Brüggemann, G.-P. (2001b). Influence of leg stiffness and its effect on myodynamic jumping performance. Journal of Electromyography and Kinesiology 11, 355–364

Becker, H.P.; Ebner, S.; Ebner, D.; Benesch, S.; Frossler, H.; Hayes, A.; Gritze, G.; Rosenbaum, D. (1999). 12-year outcome after modified Watson-Jones tenodesis for ankle instability. Clinical Orthopaedics and related research 358, 194–204

Benesch, S.; Putz, W.; Rosenbaum, D.; Becker, H. (2000). Reliability of peroneal reaction time measurements. Clinical Biomechanics 15, 21–28

Bonasera, S.J.; Nichols, T.R. (1996). Mechanical actions of heterogenic reflexes among ankle stabilizers and their interactions with plantarflexors of the cat hindlimb. Journal of Neurophysiology 75, 2050–2070

Bonato. P.; D'Alessio, T.; Knaflitz, M. (1988). A statistical method for the measurement of muscle activation intervals from surface myoelectric signal during gait. IEEE Transactions on Biomedical Engineering 45, 287–299

Brinckmann, P.; Frobin, W.; Leivseth, G. (2002). B3-Dealing with errors. In: Brinckmann, P.; Frobin, W.; Leivseth, G (Eds), Muskuloskeletal Biomechanics. Georg Thieme Verlag, Stuttgart, pp. 227–229

Cass, J.R.; Morrey, B.F.; Chao, E.Y. (1984). Three-dimensional kinematics of ankle instability following serial sectioning of lateral collateral ligaments. Foot & Ankle 5, 142–149

Caster, B.L.; Bates, B.T. (1995). The assessment of mechanical and neuromuscular response strategies during landing. Medicine and Science in Sports and Exercise 27, 736–744

Caulfield, B.M.; Garrett, M. (2002). Functional instability of the ankle: Differences in patterns of ankle and knee movement prior to and post landing in a single leg jump. International Journal of Sports Medicine 23, 64–68

Caulfield, B.M.; Garrett, M. (2004). Changes in ground reaction force during jump landing in subjects with functional instability of the ankle joint. Clinical Biomechanics 19, 617–621

Cohen, L.A.; Cohen, M.L. (1956). Arthrokinetic reflex of the knee. American Journal of Physiology. 184, 433–437

Di Fabio, R.P. (1987). Reliability of computerized surface electromyography for determining the onset of muscle activity. Physical Therapy 67, 43–48

Dufek, J.S.; Bates, B.T. (1990). The evaluation and prediction of impact forces during landings. Medicine and Science in Sports and Exercise 22, 370–377

Duncan, A.; McDonagh, M.J. (2000). Stretch reflex distinguished from pre-programmed muscle activations following landing impacts in man. Journal of Physiology 526, 457–568

Dyhre-Poulsen, P. Mosfeldt Laursen, A. (1984). Programmed electromyographic activity and negative incremental muscle stiffness in monkeys jumping downward. Journal of Physiology 350, 121–136

Dyhre-Poulsen, P.; Simonsen, E.B.; Voigt, M. (1991). Dynamic control of muscle stiffness and H reflex modulation during hopping and jumping in man. Journal of Physiology 437, 287–304

Ebig, M.; Lephart, S.M.; Burdett, R.G.; Miller, M.C.; Pincivero, D.M. (1997). The effect of sudden inversion stress on EMG activity of the peroneal and tibialis anterior muscles in the chronically unstable ankle. Journal of Orthopedy, Sports and Physical Therapy 26, 73–77

Eils, E.; Rosenbaum, D. (2003). The main function of ankle braces is to control the joint position before landing. Foot & Ankle 24, 263–268

Engeln-Müllges, G.; Reutter, F. (1991). Formelsammlung zur Numerischen Mathematik mit Turbo Pascal-Programmen. Wissenschaftsverlag Mannheim/Wien/Zürich

Flanagan, J.R.; Vetter, P.; Johansson, R.S.; Wolpert, D.M. (2003). Prediction precedes control in motor learning. Current Biology 13. 146–150

Freeman, M.A.; Dean, M.R.; Hanham, I.W. (1965). The etiology and prevention of functional instability of the foot. Journal of Bone and Joint Surgery 47, 678–685

Gauffin, H.; Tropp, H.; Odenrick, P. (1988). Effect of ankle disk training on postural control in patients with functional instability of the ankle joint. Journal of Sports Medicine 9, 141–144

Gollhofer, A.; Horstmann, G.A.; Schmidtbleicher, D.; Schönthal, D. (1990). Reproducibility of electromyographic patterns in stretch-shortening type contractions. European Journal of Applied Physiology 60, 7–14

Goodwin, P.C.; Koorts, K.; Mack, R.; Mai, S.; Morrissey, M.C.; Hooper, D.M. (1999). Reliability of leg muscle electromyography in vertical jumping. European Journal of Applied Physiology 79, 374–378

Gross, T.S.; Nelson, R.C. (1988). The shock attenuation role of the ankle during landing from a vertical jump. Medicine and Science in Sports and Exercise 20, 506–514

Grüneberg, C.; Nieuwenhuijzen, P.H.; Duysens, J. (2003). Reflex responses in the lower leg following landing impact on an inverting and non-inverting platform. Journal of Physiology 550, 985–993

Hayes, K.C. (1982). Biomechanics of postural control. Exercise and Sport Sciences Reviews 10, 363–391

Hodges, P.W.; Bui, B.H. (1996). A comparison of computer-based methods for the determination of onset of muscle contraction using electromyography. Electroencefalography & Clinical Neurophysiology 101, 511–519

Isakov, E.; Mizrahi, J.; Solzi, P.; Susak, Z.; Lotem, M. (1986). Response of the peroneal muscles to sudden inversion of the ankle during standing. International Journal of Sports Biomechanics 2, 100–109

Johnson, M.B.; Johnson, C.L. (1993). Electromyographic response of peroneal muscles in surgical and nonsurgical injured ankles during sudden inversion. Journal of Orthopedy, Sports and Physical Therapy 18, 497–501

Kadaba, M.P.; Wootten, M.E.; Gainey, J.; Cochran, G.V. (1985). Repeatability of phasic muscle activity: performance of surface and intramuscular wire electrodes in gait analysis. Journal of Orthopedic Research 3, 350–359

Kamen, G.; Caldwell, G.E. (1996). Physiology and interpretation of the electromyogram. Journal of Clinical Neurophysiology 13, 366–384

Kaminski, T.W.; Hartsell, H.D. (2002). Factors Contributing to Chronic Ankle Instability: A Strength Perspective. Journal of Athletic Training 37, 394–405

Karlsson, J.; Eriksson, B.I.; Renstrom, P.A. (1997). Subtalar ankle instability. A review. Sports Medicine 24, 337–346

Karlsson, J.; Andreasson, G.O. (1992). The effect of external ankle support in chronic lateral ankle joint instability. An electromyographic study. The American Journal of Sports Medicine 20, 257–261

Karlsson, J.; Peterson L.; Andreasson, G.; Hogfors, C. (1992). The unstable ankle, A combined EMG and Biomechanical Modeling Study. International Journal of Sports Biomechanics 8, 129–144

Katz, B. (1939). The relation between force and speed in muscular contraction. Journal of Physiology 96, 45–64

Kleinrensink, G.J.; Stoeckart, R.; Meulstee, J.; Kaulesar Sukul, D.M.; Vleeming, A.; Snijders, C.J.; van Noort, A. (1994). Lowered motor conduction velocity of the peroneal nerve after inversion trauma. Medicine and Science in Sports and Exercise 26, 877–883

Konradsen, L. (2002). Factors contributing to chronic ankle instability: Kinesthesia and joint position sense. Journal of Athletic Training 37, 381–385

Konradsen, L.; Olesen, S.; Hansen, H.M. (1998). Ankle sensorimotor control and eversion strength after acute ankle inversion injuries. The American Journal of Sports Medicine 26, 72–77

Konradsen, L.; Ravn, J.B. (1990). Ankle instability caused by prolonged peroneal reaction time. Acta Orthopaedica Scandinavica 61, 388–390

Konradsen, L.; Voigt, M.; Hojsgaard, C. (1997). Ankle inversion injuries. The role of the dynamic defense mechanism. American Journal of Sports Medicine 25, 54–58

Leanderson, J.; Bergqvist, M.; Rolf, C.; Westblad, P.; Wigelius-Roovers, S.; Wredmark, T. (1999). Early influence of an ankle sprain on objective measures of ankle joint function. A prospective randomised study of ankle brace treatment. Knee Surgery, Sports Traumatology, Arthroscopy 7, 51–58

Lephart, S.M.; Pincivero, D.M.; Giraldo, J.L.; Fu, F.H. (1997). The role of proprioception in the management and rehabilitation of athletic injuries. American Journal of Sports Medicine 25, 130–137

Liebermann, D.G.; Hoffman, J.R. (2005). Timing of preparatory landing responses as a function of availability of optic flow information. Journal of Electromyography and Kinesiology 15, 120–130

Liu, W.; Maitland, M.E.; Nigg, B.M. (2000). The effect of axial load on the in vivo anterior drawer test of the ankle joint complex. Foot & Ankle 21, 420–426

Loeb, G.E. (1995). Control implications of musculoskeletal mechanics. Book of abstracts of the Annual International Conference of the IEEE-EMBS 17, 1393–1394

Löfvenberg, R.; Kärrholm, J.; Sundelin, G.; Ahlgren, O. (1995). Prolonged reaction time in patients with chronic lateral instability of the ankle. The American Journal of Sports Medicine 23, 414–417

Lynch, S.A.; Eklund, U.; Gottlieb, D.; Renstrom, P.A.; Beynnon, B. (1996). Electromyographic latency changes in the ankle musculature during inversion moments. The American Journal of Sports Medicine 24, 362–369

Marigold, D.S.; Patla, A.E. (2002). Strategies for dynamic stability during locomotion on a slippery surface: effects of prior experience and knowledge. Journal of Neurophysiology 88: 339–353

McKinley, P.; Pedotti, A. (1992). Motor strategies in landing from a jump: the role of skill in task execution. Experimental Brain Research 90, 427–440

Mero, A.; Komi, P.V. (1986). Force-, EMG-, and elasticity velocity relationship at submaximal, maximal and supramaximal running speeds in sprinters. European Journal of Applied Physiology and Occupational Physiology 55, 553–561

Morey-Klapsing, G.; Arampatzis, A.; Brüggemann, G.P. (2004). Choosing EMG parameters: comparison of different onset determination algorithms and EMG integrals in a joint stability study. Clinical Biomechanics 19, 196–201

Moritz, C.T.; Farley, C.T. (2004). Passive dynamics change leg mechanics for an unexpected surface during human hopping. Journal of Applied Physiology 97, 1313–1322

Myers, J.B.; Riemann, B.L.; Hwang, J.H.; Fu, F.H.; Lephart, S.M. (2003). Effect of peripheral afferent alteration of the lateral ankle ligaments on dynamic stability. The American Journal of Sports Medicine 31, 498–506

Neely, F.G. (1998). Biomechanical risk factors for exercise-related lower limb injuries. Sports Medicine 26, 395–413

Nielsen, J.B. (2004). Sensorimotor integration at spinal level as a basis for muscle coordination during voluntary movement in humans. Journal of Applied Physiology 96, 1961–1967

Nieuwenhuijzen, P.H.; Gruneberg, C.; Duysens, J. (2002). Mechanically induced ankle inversion during human walking and jumping. Journal of Neuroscience Methods 112, 133–140

Patton, J.L.; Lee, W.A.; Pai, Y.C. (2000). Relative stability improves with experience in a dynamic standing task. Experimental Brain Research 135, 117–126

Pelland, L.; McKinley, P. (2004). A pattern recognition technique to characterize the differential modulation of co-activating muscles at the performer/environment interface. Journal of Electromyography and Kinesiology 14, 539–554

Riemann, B.L.; Myers, J.B.; Lephart, S.M. (2003). Comparison of the ankle, knee, hip, and trunk corrective action shown during single-leg stance on firm, foam, and multiaxial surfaces. Archives of Physical Medicine and Rehabilitation 84, 90–95

Santello, M. (2005). Review of motor control mechanisms underlying impact absorption from falls. Gait Posture 21, 85–94

Santello, M.; McDonagh, M.J. (1998). The control of timing and amplitude of EMG activity in landing movements in humans. Experimental Physiology 83, 857–874

Scheuffelen, C.; Gollhofer, A.; Lohrer, H. (1993). Neuartige funktionelle Untersuchungen zum Stabilisierungsverhalten von Sprunggelenksorthesen. Sportverletzung – Sportschaden 7, 30–36

Self, B.P.; Paine, D. (2001). Ankle biomechanics during four landing techniques. Medicine and Science in Sports and Exercise 33, 1338–1344

Seligson, D.; Gassman, J.; Pope, M. (1980). Ankle instability: Evaluation of the lateral ligaments. The American Journal of Sports Medicine 8, 39–42

Siegler, S.; Wang, D.; Plasha, E.; Berman, T. (1994). Technique for in vivo measurement of the three-dimensional kinematics and laxity characteristics of the ankle joint complex. Journal of orthopaedic research 12, 421–431

Stacoff, A.; Kaelin, X.; Stuessi, E.; Segesser, B. (1990). Die Torsionsbewegung des Fußes beim Landen nach einem Sprung. Zeitschrift für Orthopädie und Ihre Grenzgebiete 128, 213–217

Stacoff, A.; Reinschmidt, C.; Nigg, B.M.; van den Bogert, A.J.; Lundberg, A.; Denoth, J.; Stüssi, E. (2000). Effects of foot orthoses on skeletal motion during running. Clinical Biomechanics 15, 54–64

Thompson, H.W.; McKinley, P.A. (1995). Landing from a jump: the role of vision when landing from known and unknown heights. Neuro Report 6, 581–584

Tomberg, C.; Levarlet-Joye, H.; Desmedt, J.E. (1991). Reaction times recording methods: reliability and EMG analysis of patterns of motor commands. Electroencefalography & Clinical Neurophysiology 81, 269–278

Tropp, H.; Askling, J.; Gillquist, J. (1985). Prevention of ankle sprains. American Journal of Sports Medicine 13, 259–262

Tropp, H.; Odenrick, P. (1988). Postural control in single-limb stance. Journal of Orthopaedic Research 6, 833–839

Vaes, P.; Van Gheluwe, B.; Duquet, W. (2001). Control of acceleration during sudden ankle supination in people with unstable ankles. Journal of Orthopedy, Sports and Physical Therapy 31, 741–752

Verhagen, E.A.; van Mechelen, W.; de Vente, W. (2000). The effect of preventive measures on the incidence of ankle sprains. Clinical Journal of Sport Medicine 10, 291–296

Wagner, H.; Blickhan, R. (2003). Stabilizing function of antagonistic neuromusculoskeletal systems: an analytical investigation. Biological Cybernetics 89, 71–79

Winter, D.A. (1984). Pathologic gait diagnosis with computer-averaged electromyographic profiles. Arch Phys Med Rehabil 65, 393–398

Wittenburg, J. (1977). Dynamics of systems of rigid bodies. B.G. Teubner Stuttgart

Wright, I.C.; Neptune, R.R.; van den Bogert, A.J.; Nigg, B.M. (2000). The influence of foot positioning on ankle sprains. Journal of Biomechanics 33, 513–519

Yang, J.F.; Winter, D.A. (1983). Electromyography reliability in maximal and submaximal isometric contractions. Archives of physical medicine and rehabilitation. 64, 417–420

Zhou, S.; Lawson, D.L.; Morrison, W.E.; Fairweather, I. (1995). Electromechanical delay in isometric muscle contractions evoked by voluntary, reflex and electrical stimulation. European Journal of Applied Physiology 70, 138–145

Curriculum Vitae

Gaspar Maximilian Gabriel Morey Klapsing was born in Essen (Germany) in 1971. In 1978 he moved to Palma de Mallorca (Spain) with his family. In 1989 he moved to Valencia (Spain) where he studied physical education at the University of Valencia (Institut Valencià d'educació física). From February 1994 to February 1995 he enjoyed a grant from the Polytechnic University of Valencia at the IBV (Institut de Biomecànica de València) in the group of sport biomechanics. In 1994 he got his diploma in physical education (Licenciatura en educación física) and in 1995 the certificate for teaching aptitude (CAP: Certificat d'aptitud pedagògica). This same year he visited a course in neurophysiological techniques in clinical practice at the University of the Balearic Islands.

Short time later he moved to Cologne (Germany) where he joined the research group led by Prof. Brüggemann at the German Sport University Cologne and accomplished his doctorate studies. In 1997 he became scientific assistant at the Institute for Athletics and Gymnastics. In 2001 the research group moved to the institute for Biomechanics (now Institute for Biomechanics and Orthopaedics). Later this year he became scientific co-worker of the institute.

In the last years he participated in several research projects mainly related to footwear, sport materials and movement analysis. His main interests in basic research are in the fields of joint stabilisation, muscle mechanics and more recently motor control as well.

He authored and co-authored more than 50 papers and abstracts in international peer reviewed journals and congress proceedings. In addition he translated a book on infantile gymnastics and several technical texts (e.g. DIN norms on sport surfaces) from the German language into Spanish.

Schriftenreihe zur Biomechanik des muskulo-skelettalen Systems

Gert-Peter Brüggemann (Hrsg.)

▪ Band 1

Niehoff, Anja
Belastung und Adaptation der Epiphysenfuge

Eine prospektive Untersuchung zur Anpassung biomechanischer, morphologischer und biochemischer Parameter der distalen Femurepiphysenfuge an mechanische Belastung.
Köln 2003. 185 Seiten, 68 z. T. farb. Abb., 17 Tab.
ISBN 3-89001-603-0   € 34,00

▪ Band 2

Potthast, Wolfgang
Stoßübertragung über das Knie und muskuläre Gelenkkopplung

Köln 2005. 120 Seiten, 33 Abb., 9 Tab.
ISBN 3-89001-604-9   € 34,00

▪ Band 3

Morey-Klapsing, Gaspar Maximilian Gabriel
Stabilisation of the foot and ankle complex: Proactive and reactive responses to disturbances in the frontal plane

Köln 2005. 116 Seiten, 25 z. T. farb. Abb., 13 Tab.
ISBN 3-89001-605-7   € 34,00